The Baby Development Test

A step-by-step guide to your baby's development from birth to 5 years

Dr Dorothy Einon

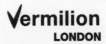
LONDON

1 3 5 7 9 10 8 6 4 2

First published in the United Kingdom in 2006 by Vermilion
an imprint of Ebury Publishing
Random House UK Limited, Random House, 20 Vauxhall Bridge Road, London SW1V 2SA

Random House Australia (Pty) Limited
20 Alfred Street, Milsons Point, Sydney, New South Wales 2061, Australia

Random House New Zealand Limited
18 Poland Road, Glenfield, Auckland 10, New Zealand

Random House (Pty) Limited
Isle of Houghton, Corner of Boundary Road & Carse O'Gowrie, Houghton 2198, South Africa

Random House Publishers India Private Limited
301 World Trade Tower, Hotel Intercontinental Grand Complex,
Barakhamba Lane, New Delhi 110 001, India

Random House UK Limited Reg. No. 954009
www.randomhouse.co.uk
Papers used by Vermilion are natural, recyclable products
made from wood grown in sustainable forests.

A CIP catalogue record is available for this book from the British Library.

ISBN: 009191051X
ISBN 13: 9780091910518 (from January 2007)

Designed and typeset by seagulls.net

Printed and bound in Great Britain by Mackays of Chatham plc, Chatham, Kent

Copies are available at special rates for bulk orders.
Contact the sales development team on 020 7840 8487
or visit www.booksforpromotions.co.uk for more information.

Contents

Introduction

This book uses a series of specially developed tests to examine your child's development over the first five years. In the first chapter we look at physical and mental development in the early years. These are not intelligence tests (it is extremely hard to predict intelligence from the behavioural development of babies), but rather tell you what the average baby, toddler and child can do at certain ages. The second chapter looks at cognitive skills – thinking, learning and memory – and the third chapter looks at language skills. The fourth chapter addresses the child's knowledge of himself and others – and his independence, the fifth chapter looks at temperament and the final chapter examines your parenting skills.

The tests presented here are based on those developed by psychologists who study child development. They include simple questions and answers; checklists, which list various behaviours in the typical order they develop in the average child; and some classic experiments that psychologists have used to show that a child is able to understand a certain concept. Research in the United States has shown that those who work in childcare provide a more stimulating environment for the children in their care if they have received some training in child development. The aim of these tests is to give parents that advantage: to help them to know their child's capabilities so that they are in a better position to play to their strengths and help them succeed.

Not all children develop at the same rate: a child who reaches one motor milestone (like holding her head up or rolling over) early tends to meet other milestones sooner than other children of the same age. The same is true for those children who are late reaching these milestones. Motor development – the ability to move and control our bodies – depends on the maturity of the brain and body mechanisms, and this in turn means that those who reach milestones early have brains that are maturing faster than those who reach them late. Just as we would not consider that those reaching sexual maturity earlier are likely to be more sexy, or that breasts that start to mature earliest will ultimately be bigger, we should not worry that a child who is slow to reach her milestones is somehow not as bright. Except at the extremes (where damage to the brain, or errors in development, affect both motor and intellectual functions), slow starters catch up.

All children receive a boost in their capabilities when they first become mobile. They take a sudden leap forward because movement opens up their world. Not only are they able to explore when the mood takes them but they naturally put together sequences of actions: crawl across the room and look behind the chair; crawl to the cupboard and get out the bricks; retrieve the ball and push it in the shape sorter. This challenges them and boosts their capabilities. In turn, children who are late creeping, crawling and walking start to fall behind. But it is a temporary setback. Like all babies, late crawlers take that leap ahead once they start to move. Research suggests that although early crawlers/walkers jump ahead, they do not maintain their lead. Late crawlers catch up when they start to move about and within months it is impossible to tell them apart.

Before doing the tests in this book, bear in mind that they do not measure intelligence, nor do they predict school attainment. Babies cannot solve mathematical or logic problems, tell us how a mortgage works, nor copy a pattern we have made with bricks. What they *can* do is reach for things we offer them, listen and understand some of the things that we say to them, and try to communicate with us. At the earliest stages this is all that we can test. If motor skills were closely related to intelligence our universities would be staffed by ex-footballers and our playing fields and running tracks filled with young lawyers and scientists. Nor is the precocious acquisition of language a foolproof guide to intelligence: by some accounts Einstein, who was probably one of the cleverest men who ever lived, did not speak until he was almost two years old.

In other words, the sorts of tests you are about to do are only marginally predictive of later intelligence tests. It is only when children have developed the capacity to do the things that school-age children and adults do (which is around the time they start school), that tests can be designed that are able to predict adult skills and abilities and long-term academic success.

What preschool development tests can tell you is how your child 'measures up' and this helps you to understand how to encourage and stimulate development. It also lets you know where she is likely to be in a month or two (which can help you plan ahead). Maturity does not occur in a vacuum, but is influenced by the environment a child finds herself in. No amount of practice will perfect a skill much before time, but if the timing is right, practice helps perfect a skill and those who are enriched by their experiences are likely to do better than those who are not.

One other thing we need to keep in mind is the meaning of the word 'average'. Average is the middle, so when we say the average six-month-old can do something, we mean that half the babies of this age will NOT be able to do it yet, and the other half will do somewhat better. Remember that for many things we should count development as starting from conception, not birth, so babies who are born early for dates are likely to be late. The onset of smiling, facial expressions, mobility and coordination are examples. In premature babies these bear more relationship to their due date than their birth date.

Top Tips

1. A child should always be encouraged to believe 'I can if I try.' Even in something like mathematics that requires instruction, belief works as well as extra tuition.

2. Love is a child's birthright. Children should always know they are loved for who they are, not what they can do.

3. A child who knows he is loved is a happier child – and happier children find it easier to learn.

4. Stress is the enemy of progress and so we should try to reduce stress as far as we can.

5. Children should feel free to express their opinions.

6. Children should be encouraged to express, manipulate and evaluate ideas.

7. Children feel more secure when discipline is firm but fair, when there are clearly defined limits and expectations that they will adhere to.

8. Parents should help children find problems as well as helping them to solve them.

9. Children should be provided with a safe and stimulating environment.

10. Distractions should be kept to a minimum – the TV should not be on all the time, and noise levels should be kept down.

Chapter 1
The Developmental Tests

The developmental tests look at a wide range of skills that most children develop in the early years of life, including physical skills, social skills and coordination of movement, play and language. The overall score gives a rough indication of whether or not your child is 'on target'. Remember, nothing is very precise at this age and children change rapidly. So, for example, although the average child is unsteady on his feet until he is 14–15 months old, a few children walk five months earlier than this and some perfectly normal children will not walk for another five months. The age at which children walk is not related to intelligence or indeed to physical prowess.

Children's progression is rarely gradual. Although by and large children's scores are increasing month on month, their progression is often composed of a short leap followed by a slow consolidation. In other words, one week he seems to be growing up in a rush, but then in the following weeks progression is much more gradual.

HOW TO SCORE THE TESTS
1 for each a, 2 for each b, 3 for each c.
Then add up the numbers and see 'Interpreting the Scores'.

The Baby Development Test: 6–12 Months

1. Does your child

a) Turn his head away when he doesn't want food? ○

b) Lift his arms to be picked up? ○

c) Play pat-a-cake or wave goodbye? ○

2. Can your child

a) Grab a toy you hand him? ○

b) Drop a toy on purpose? ○

c) Stack two cups or two bricks? ○

3. Does your child

a) Find opening little doors in his toys too difficult? ○

b) Use his hand to push open a little door? ○

c) Use a finger to push open a little door? ○

4. Does your child

a) Use his hand to try to pick up little bits of food? ○

b) Use a finger and thumb to pick up peas? ○

c) Use his finger and thumb to pick up and put down things? ○

5. Does your child

a) Enjoy songs like 'This little piggy' or 'Ride a cock horse'? ○

b) Put out his foot in readiness for 'This little piggy'? ○

c) Do some of the actions for a song like 'Pat-a-cake, pat-a-cake'? ○

6. How many things can your child tell you?

a) One sign (a movement or noise that tells you 'pick me up', 'no', 'look', 'do it again', etc). ○

b) Two or more signs. ○

c) One or more words or animal noises (even if not very clear). ○

7. Does your child

a) Ignore a toy he drops? ○

b) Look for a toy he drops? ○

c) Intentionally drop toys and watch where they go? ○

8. Can your child

a) Have a babble conversation with you? ○

b) Look where you look? ○

c) Imitate an action, such as pretending to drink from a toy cup? ○

9. Can your child

a) Smack things with an open hand? ○

b) Prod things with a finger? ○

c) Point to show you things? ○

10. Does your child

a) Treat all toys in the same way?

b) Mostly bang and suck, but cuddle his teddy or knock over a brick tower?

c) Do what is expected: open doors, press buttons, stack cups?

11. Does your child

a) Look away when you cover a toy with a cloth?

b) Look under the cloth if part of the toy is peeping out?

c) Lift the cloth to find the hidden toy?

12. Does your child

a) Know his name?

b) Look for his daddy when you ask, 'Where's Daddy?'?

c) Use a 'name' for someone he loves (even if it's only a noise)?

13. Does your child

a) Vocalise pleasure and displeasure?

b) Stop doing something when you say 'No'?

c) Try to imitate words such as 'Mama', 'Dada' or 'Woof woof'?

14. Will your child

a) Reach persistently for a block that is out of reach?

b) Imitate the way you stir and rattle a spoon in a cup? ○
c) Put a round block into a round hole? ○

15. Does your child

a) Imitate what you do if you bang your hand on the table? ○
b) Push or 'brum' a small car along? ○
c) Hug and kiss a favourite teddy? ○

INTERPRETING THE SCORES

❑ The average six-month-old will not be able to do everything on the list but should be able to get an 'a' for the majority of questions. He may even get an occasional 'b' but probably not 'c' scores. *Expected score in the region of 12–17.*

❑ The average nine-month-old may still have a few 'a' scores but should be getting more 'b' scores. *Expected score of 25–30.*

❑ The average 12-month-old is expected to gain mostly 'c' scores with some 'b' scores. *Expected score of 34–36.*

The Toddler Development Test: 12–18 Months

1. Can your child clap his hands, wave bye-bye and indicate he wants to be lifted up?

a) No, none of these. ○
b) One of these. ○
c) Two or more of these. ○

2. Can your child

a) Put an object into a container?

b) Build a tower of two cubes?

c) Build a tower of three cubes?

3. Can your child

a) Find a toy he sees you hide?

b) Search in several different places for a toy you have hidden?

c) Find a toy you have moved when he is not looking?

4. How many words does your child use?

a) One word (even if it is not very clear).

b) Three words.

c) Six plus words.

5. Does your child

a) Use and explore toys by playing with them in different ways (banging some, cuddling others)?

b) Experiment with different actions when trying to solve problems (such as twisting his hand in different ways when trying to get a shape into his shape sorter)?

c) Sometimes appear to have found the solution without obviously experimenting?

6. Can your child
a) Imitate an action you show him? ○
b) 'Brum' a car? ○
c) Feed a doll? ○

7. If you take two objects and slide one underneath a cloth, then lift a cloth and lay it over the other, does your child
a) Not look for either object? ○
b) First look for the object you put the cloth over? ○
c) First look for the object you put under the cloth? ○

8. Can your child
a) Put together an action and a sound (for example, point and say 'Woof woof')? ○
b) Put together an action and word (point and say 'Bus')? ○
c) Put together two words? ○

9. Does your child point
a) To show you things? ○
b) To show things you have asked him to show you? ○
c) At pictures in a book? ○

10. Is your child able to identify a picture by pointing at items you name?

a) No.

b) Yes.

c) Yes, by pointing *and* by naming (even if the word isn't clear).

11. When your child plays with his farm animals is he

a) Unable to group them together in any systematic way?

b) Able to put all the cows in one place and all the sheep in another?

c) Able to put the mothers with their babies?

12. Is your child

a) Unable to follow a command with gestures (if you point to emphasise what you want)?

b) Able to follow a command with gestures (when you point to emphasise what you want)?

c) Able to follow a one-step command without gestures?

13. Can your child

a) Hold, bite and chew a biscuit?

b) Feed himself with a spoon – spilling a lot?

c) Feed himself with a spoon – spilling very little?

14. Does your child

a) Put his hands on his cup when drinking?

b) Drink from a cup with assistance?

c) Manage a cup without assistance?

15. If given a crayon and paper does your child

a) Hold the crayon but not draw with it?

b) Scribble a little if encouraged?

c) Start scribbling?

INTERPRETING THE SCORES

❑ The average 12-month-old will not be able to do everything here but should be able to get an 'a' for the majority of questions. He may even get an occasional 'b' but probably not any 'c' scores. *Expected score in the region of 13–19.*

❑ The average 15-month-old should be getting more 'b' scores. *Expected score in the region of 25–30.*

❑ The average 18-month-old is expected to gain mostly 'b's with some 'c' scores. *Expected score of 34–38.*

The Toddler Development Test: 18–24 Months

1. When playing with a ball can your child

a) Roll it to an adult? ○

b) Throw or kick it without falling over? ○

c) Throw the ball into a basket placed 60 cm away? ○

2. When feeding himself does your child

a) Use fingers and a spoon – spilling quite a lot of food from the spoon? ○

b) Manage to control the spoon – spilling food only occasionally? ○

c) Use a spoon and pusher or fork together? ○

3. When your child wants something he cannot name does he

a) Use gestures to make wants known – for example, pointing to a toy on the shelf? ○

b) Point to distant objects to indicate he needs them? ○

c) Pull you to come with him to look for the thing he needs? ○

4. Does your child understand when asked

a) Not to do something? ○

b) To give you the toy by name that you have neither pointed to or looked at, e.g. 'Give me the crayon'? ○

c) To fetch a toy that neither of you can see, from a place you name such as another room, a drawer or cupboard, e.g. 'Go and get your coat from the hook', 'Go and get your bike from the kitchen'?   ○

5. Can your child

a) Name one or two objects?   ○
b) Use words to make his wants known, e.g. 'Gimme'?   ○
c) Ask for things by name, 'Gimme teddy', 'Me juice'?   ○

6. When your child talks does he

a) Mostly babble but include one or two clear words?   ○
b) Use 20 or more clear words?   ○
c) Put two words together to form a simple factual sentence, 'Daddy gone', 'Bye-bye bus'?   ○

7. When looking at a book does your child

a) Recognise two or three pictures of objects?   ○
b) Use actions with pictures – such as pretending to pat the dog?   ○
c) Listen as you read a sentence without trying to turn the page?   ○

8. Does your child ever

a) Hug and kiss a doll or teddy? ○

b) Pretend to feed a doll or put a teddy to bed? ○

c) String together two 'pretend' sequences, e.g. feed a doll and then pretend to wash its face or put a doll to bed and cover it with a blanket? ○

9. If given a crayon and paper will your child

a) Start to scribble? ○

b) Scribble-draw circles and lines? ○

c) Succeed in copying a line and try to copy a circle? ○

10. Does your child

a) Look in the right place for toys that have rolled out of sight? ○

b) Look systematically for toys he cannot find – search the appropriate cupboard, etc? ○

c) Remember where a toy has been left? ○

11. Can your child

a) Imitate a simple action – copy when you tap a pencil, for example? ○

b) Imitate a more complex action such as reading a book or kissing teddies goodnight? ○

c) Imitate a single domestic activity – such as dusting, sweeping or washing? ⚬

12. When getting undressed does your child

a) Cooperate by lifting arms or holding out a foot? ⚬
b) Take off his own shoes and socks? ⚬
c) Remove simple articles of clothing such as pants or vests? ⚬

13. When your child plays with his farm animals is he able to

a) Put all the cows in one place and all the sheep in another? ⚬
b) Put the mothers with their babies? ⚬
c) Make families of animals: mother, father and baby? ⚬

14. If you place a mark on your child's forehead and then sit with him looking in the mirror does he

a) Pat and smile at his reflection in the mirror? ⚬
b) Rub the mark on his head rather than on the reflection? ⚬
c) Rub the mark on his head *and* recognise familiar adults (including himself) in photographs? ⚬

INTERPRETING THE SCORES

❑ The average 18-month-old will not be able to do everything here but should be able to get an 'a' for the majority of questions. He may even get an occasional 'b' but probably not 'c' scores. *Expected score in the region of 13–19.*

❑ The average 21-month-old should be getting more 'b' scores. *Expected score of 25–30.*

❑ The average 24-month-old is expected to gain mostly 'b's with some 'c' scores. *Expected score of 34–38.*

The Toddler Development Test: 2–3 Years

1. Can your child
a) Jump off the bottom step of the stairs? ○
b) Alternate feet when going upstairs? ○
c) Jump off the second step of the stairs? ○

2. Can your child
a) Kick a ball without falling over? ○
b) Run after a ball? ○
c) Catch a large ball thrown from a metre away? ○

3. Can your child
a) Feed himself with a spoon – without making much mess? ○
b) Use a spoon and fork – or pusher – to feed himself? ○
c) Use a spoon and fork (or pusher) skilfully? ○

4. Does your child
a) Let you know when he needs the toilet? ○

b) Take down his pants and go to the toilet alone?   ○ ○
c) Go to the toilet, use tissue and flush?   ○

5. Does your child
a) Ask for things by name?   ○
b) Carry on simple conversations about past experiences?   ○
c) Describe what he wants in detail?   ○

6. Does your child
a) Cooperate when you wash him?   ○
b) Wash and dry his own hands?   ○
c) Brush his teeth – providing you direct and encourage him?   ○

7. Does your child
a) Need help when getting dressed?   ○
b) Manage to put on some items, e.g. pants, socks?   ○
c) Dress and undress without help, except for fastenings
    and awkward items of clothing?   ○

9. Will your child
a) Amuse himself when you are busy?   ○
b) Start to play with toys when left alone?   ○
c) Play outside if you watch him from the house?   ○

9. Can your child
a) Copy a line you have drawn?
b) Copy a circle?
c) Draw a rudimentary person – a head, eyes and perhaps legs?

10. When with children of about the same age does your child
a) Play alongside them and sometimes share toys but rarely, if ever, join in their games?
b) Play with one other child?
c) Play cooperatively with more than one child?

11. Does your child's make-believe play include
a) Simple activities – pretending to be asleep or to feed a teddy?
b) Quite elaborate domestic activities – such as cooking dinner at his stove and pretending to eat it?
c) Pretending to be someone else (such as Father Christmas) with appropriate actions (delivering toys from a sack)?

12. Does your child
a) Recognise familiar objects in pictures?
b) Recognise photos of familiar people?
c) Recognise tiny details in pictures?

13. Can your child

a) Follow simple directions, e.g. 'Get your coat'?

b) Follow directions that include the prepositions 'on' or 'in', e.g. 'Put the toys in the box', 'Put the cup on the table'?

c) Fetch two or three objects you name from another room?

14. Can your child

a) Match one object with another of the same (put a toy pig with another toy pig)?

b) AND say which pig is big and which small?

c) AND tell which pig is heavy and which light?

15. Can your child

a) Put two words together, 'Gimme juice', 'Bye-bye Daddy'?

b) Put three words together, 'Daddy gone work'?

c) Use pronouns (I, me, my) and plurals (cats, spoons)?

INTERPRETING THE SCORES

❑ The average two-year-old will not be able to do everything here but should be able to get an 'a' for the majority of questions. He may even get an occasional 'b' but probably not 'c' scores. *Expected score in the region of 13–19.*

❑ The average two-and-a-half-year-old should be getting more 'b' scores. *Expected score of 25–30.*

❑ The average three-year-old is expected to gain mostly 'b's with some 'c' scores. *Expected score of 34–38.*

The Preschool Development Test: 3–4 Years

1. Does your child
a) Ask for things by name, 'Milk', 'Juice'? ○
b) Describe in detail what he wants, 'A biscuit with a smiley face'? ○
c) Do both of the above and also continuously ask why? ○

2. When going up and down stairs does your child
a) Go up and down stairs leading with the same foot? ○
b) Alternate feet going up but lead with one foot on the way down? ○
c) Go up AND down alternating feet? ○

3. Can your child
a) Throw a small ball or beanbag into a basket 60 cm away? ○
b) Catch a large ball thrown from 120 cm away? ○
c) Run and kick a ball without first stopping? ○

4. At the table is your child able to
a) Use two implements (such as spoon and fork) together when eating? ○

b) Use a knife to spread butter or jam (although perhaps not skilfully)? ○

c) Use a knife and fork skilfully? ○

5. Can your child

a) Manage a cup well? ○

b) Drink from an almost-full cup without spilling? ○

c) Pour milk from a jug or bottle onto his cereal? ○

6. When playing does your child

a) Use objects inappropriately – such as using a cloth as a hat, or a chair as a car? ○

b) Pretend that something is there when it is not – such as holding an imaginary wheel when pretending to drive? ○

c) Pretend to be something or someone else? ○

7. Does your child

a) Wash and dry his hands without help? ○

b) Wash his face – but still need help with neck and ears? ○

c) Brush his teeth by himself? ○

9. Can your child

a) Copy a circle you have drawn? ○

b) Draw a person with legs and a head? ○

c) Draw a person with head, face, body, arms or legs? ○

9. The following questions are about your child's understanding of concepts

a) When asked, is he able to hide a toy *under* a cloth? ○

b) If asked, could he bring you the brick *nearest* the radiator? ○

c) If asked, could he put a sweet *last* in a line? ○

10. Can your child

a) Get somebody from another room when asked? ○

b) Greet familiar adults without being reminded to do so ('Say hi to Nanna')? ○

c) Contribute to adult conversation? ○

11. Does your child

a) Talk about how he is feeling? ○

b) Ask for help when he needs it? ○

c) Comfort you when you are unhappy or unwell? ○

12. Does your child

a) Dance to music? ○

b) Sing and dance to music? ○

c) Repeat all or part of rhymes, songs and dances when asked? ○

13. Does your child

a) Say 'please' and 'thank you' if reminded? ○

b) Often say 'please' and 'thank you' without being reminded? ○

c) Say 'sorry' without being reminded? ○

14. When speaking does your child use

a) The past tense, 'It rained', 'I walked'? ○

b) Auxiliary verbs, 'I am walking', 'I do like honey'? ○

c) Conjunctions such as 'and' and 'but' when linking events
    or statements, 'You think so BUT I don't', 'Milly is here
    AND we are going out'? ○

INTERPRETING THE SCORES

❑ The average three-year-old will not be able to do everything here
  but should be able to get an 'a' for the majority of questions. He
  may even get an occasional 'b' but probably not 'c' scores.
  Expected score in the region of 13–19.

❑ The average three-and-a-half-year-old should be getting more 'b'
  scores. *Expected score of 25–30.*

❑ The average four-year-old is expected to gain mostly 'b's with
  some 'c' scores. *Expected score of 34–38.*

The Preschool Development Test: 4–5 Years

1. Can your child
a) Point to 10 different body parts? ○
b) Pick up a specified number (1–5) of objects when asked? ○
c) Name five or more letters of the alphabet? ○

2. Can your child
a) Put on his mittens? ○
b) Unbutton his coat? ○
c) Fasten a car seat belt? ○

3. Can your child
a) Stand on one foot for 4–5 seconds? ○
b) Hop on one foot five times? ○
c) Stand on one foot (with eyes closed) for 10 seconds? ○

4. Can your child
a) Jump on the spot with both feet? ○
b) March? ○
c) Skip? ○

5. Can your child
a) Tell you about something that has just happened? ○

b) Carry out a series of three directions? ◌

c) Talk about the experiences of the day without undue prompting? ◌

6. When talking can your child

a) Talk in sentences but still sometimes leave out words, 'Mummy give baby milk'? ◌

b) Use correct grammatical sentences, 'I went shopping with Mummy'? ◌

c) Put together a 3–4 sequence story? ◌

7. When you build a tower of three bricks can your child say

a) Which brick is the highest? ◌

b) Which brick is the lowest? ◌

c) Which brick is in the middle? ◌

8. When instructed is your child able to

a) Place a teddy bear *under,* then *next to,* and finally *on top of* the bed? ◌

b) Select the *largest* soft toy from a group, say which is the *tallest* tree, and which plate contains the *most* cakes? ◌

c) Say which plate has the *fewest* cakes, and when you make a line of toys which is the *first* and which the *last* in the *queue*? ◌

9. Does your child

a) Use a spoon and, occasionally, a pusher or fork? ○

b) Use a knife to spread butter? ○

c) Use a knife and fork well? ○

10. Can your child cut paper

a) In a straight line? ○

b) In a curved line? ○

c) Around shapes? ○

11. If you show him can your child

a) Fold paper in half? ○

b) Fold paper in quarters? ○

c) Fold paper twice on the diagonal? ○

12. Can your child

a) Run in a straight line? ○

b) Run changing direction without stopping? ○

c) Pick up a ball from the ground while running? ○

13. Can your child stand on one foot for

a) Fewer than four seconds? ○

b) 4–8 seconds? ○

c) More than eight seconds? ○

14. Is your child able to

a) Jump off the second step of the stairs with feet together? ◌

b) AND walk up and down stairs with feet alternating? ◌

c) AND skip? ◌

15. When speaking does your child use

a) Auxiliary verbs, 'I am walking', 'I do like honey'? ◌

b) Conjunctions such as 'and' and 'but' between sentences, 'You think so BUT I don't', 'Milly is here AND we are going out'? ◌

c) Connectives such as 'although' between sentences, 'I will, ALTHOUGH I don't want to', 'I will, EVEN IF you don't want me to'? ◌

INTERPRETING THE SCORES

❑ The average four-year-old will not be able to do everything here but should be able to get an 'a' for the majority of questions. He may even get an occasional 'b' but probably not 'c' scores. *Expected score in the region of 13–19.*

❑ The average four-and-a-half-year-old should be getting more 'b' scores. *Expected score of 25–30.*

❑ The average five-year-old is expected to gain mostly 'b's with some 'c' scores. *Expected score of 34–38.*

What Influences Physical Development?

GENES

As a rough guide you can calculate a boy's adult height by adding his father's height to his mother's height and adding 15 cm (six inches) then dividing by two; a girl's height is roughly calculated by adding her father's height to her mother's height and taking away 15 cm (six inches) before dividing by two.

Parents' weight also predicts the child's adult weight. The tendency to become overweight runs in families: a child is more likely to be overweight if both his parents are overweight than if one parent is, and more likely to be overweight if one parent is overweight than if neither are. There is also some indication that anorexia might run in families. By no means every child that lives on chips and chocolate becomes overweight, nor do all plump babies grow up to be plump adults, nor all skinny babies and children remain skinny for the rest of their lives.

DIET

Diet influences eventual height, weight and, to some extent, behaviour. Although many children in developed countries eat the wrong foods they are rarely, if ever, undernourished (except as a consequence of illness) which means they will probably grow to a normal height. The high levels of fat and sugar in their diets mean that some children are overweight.

In the UK almost two million schoolchildren are overweight, and of these about 700,000 are obese. Over 25% of girls and 20% of boys are overweight. About 160,000 British children have high blood pressure and cholesterol, over 4,000 have Type 2 diabetes and 58,000 have bad glucose tolerance.

Children are less physically active at school and more likely to sit and watch TV or play computer games than play outside with other children. Because overweight children are less likely to exercise (it takes more effort and gives less pleasure if the child is heavy), and more likely to be bullied or teased, they often have lower self-esteem which, in turn, may encourage comfort eating, which only exacerbates the problem.

If your child is slightly overweight, simple changes to your lifestyle will make a difference:

❑ Eating five portions of fruit and vegetables every day.

❑ Drinking water or fruit juice rather than fizzy drinks.

❑ Avoiding ready-prepared meals where possible.

❑ Limiting 'junk' food such as crisps and sweets to occasional treats.

❑ Encouraging children to play with other children.

❑ Walking rather than using the car.

❑ Finding exercise your child enjoys, such as trampolining, dance classes or swimming lessons.

EXERCISE

Children are naturally active – especially when they have the space to play and access to groups of children. Under these conditions children probably do not need encouragement to run and jump. It is because we feel it is unsafe to play outside, and have much smaller families, that children often lack the opportunity to give in to their natural tendency to exercise. Since sitting and watching rather than doing is a relatively recent phenomenon in childhood it is uncertain whether there are long-term effects on growth and development, although many experts believe this lack of exercise may lead to long-term obesity.

HEALTH

Serious and prolonged illness can cause stunted growth, and if illness is painful it can distract a child from learning.

 # What Influences Cognitive/Social Development?

The following environmental factors are known to influence measured intelligence in children. Note, however, that most of the influences co-exist with poverty (single parents and those who had limited schooling are likely to be relatively poor) which may be causal here. Children tend to have a lower-measure IQ if:

1. The child's mother has a history of mental illness.

2. The mother suffers from serious anxiety.

3. The mother has rigid attitudes, beliefs and values concerning her child's development.

4. There are relatively few positive interactions between mother and child.

5. The mother left school without qualifications.

6. The main breadwinner has an unskilled occupation.

7. There are more than four children in the family.

8. The child has suffered at least 20 stressful events in childhood.

9. The father does not live with the family.

10. The child is a member of a minority group – especially one subjected to prejudice.

The Motor Checklists

The checklists below follow the child's physical and skill development over the first five years. They are based on a number of checklists that have been compiled by developmental psychologists who recorded the progress of groups of young children from birth to age five, and by checking what a cross sample of children could do at particular ages. The tests reflect the order in which skills develop and can tell us what the average child does at a certain age. Most of us do not have average children. You will almost certainly find that your child does not do things in exactly the order given here, and that they never do some things on the lists. For example, some babies never crawl and a few walk before they can stand.

Girls develop a little faster than boys – for example, they develop fine finger skills a little faster – and children of African origin a little faster than those of European origin. Again this is what the average child does. There is a good deal more variation amongst girls and amongst boys than there is between girls and boys. The same goes for ethnic differences. One rule that does seem to hold is that those who race up the list in the first months (the fast developers) tend to reach all their physical milestones early, and those who start in a more leisurely fashion continue in this way. Another rule is that speed does not predict ultimate skill. There is no evidence that those who walk at nine months go on to become athletes, or that those who do not walk until they are 21 months old do badly at sports. You will probably find that the speed at which your child develops mobility is related to the speed at which he learns to control his hands. There is little correlation between early development and later skill although by the time the child is five you should be able to pick out those with exceptional skill.

The mobility and climbing checklist

Although motor development does not follow an absolutely pre-defined order, it matures in a fairly predictable sequence. All babies sit before they stand and pull themselves up to stand before they walk (although a few hurl themselves forward before they have learned to stand alone without support, the momentum of their forward movement keeps the child balanced until they stop). Not all babies crawl before they walk, and the increased use of toddle trucks and baby walkers, together with mothers' reluctance to put babies down on their stomachs, has led to a decline in the number of babies who crawl.

The motor control sequence starts for all children at the head and moves down the body, and from the centre of the body moves out. The mouth is controlled before the neck, the neck before the back and the upper back before the lower back. The arms are controlled before the legs, the shoulders before the lower arm, the arm before the hand and the hand before the fingers. The checklist below places the child's motor capability more or less in order. Simply tick the items until they no longer apply to your child. The age at which the average child reaches these motor milestones is given on page 41.

1. His knees are flexed under his body when he lies on his tummy.

2. He can hold his head upright and steady for a few seconds.

3. His back is rounded when he is in a sitting position.

4. His head lags behind his body if he is pulled by his wrists into a sitting position.

5. He kicks and waves his arms when lying on his back. ⚪

6. He lifts his head when lying on his tummy. ⚪

7. When on his tummy his hips are flat, knees extended and arms flexed. ⚪

8. He can hold his head up when sitting, but his head tends to fall forward. ⚪

9. He supports his head with his arm when lying on his tummy. ⚪

10. He holds his head steady and upright while sitting on your lap. ⚪

11. His head still lags a little when he is pulled by his arms to a sitting position. ⚪

12. He can now raise his head 45 degrees from the floor when on his stomach. ⚪

13. If he is on your knee and his back is supported he holds himself quite firmly. ⚪

14. He can roll from his stomach to his side. ⚪

15. There is now almost no head lag when he is pulled by the arms into a sitting position. ⚪

16. He can raise his head and chest 90 degrees from the floor when lying on his stomach. ⚪

17. He splashes with arms and legs when in the bath. ⚪

18. His head no longer lags when he is pulled upright by his arms. ⚪

19. His back is now quite straight when he is in a sitting position. ○

20. He can roll from his stomach to his back when lying down. ○

21. He puts his feet to his mouth when lying on his back. ○

22. He can lift his chest and upper abdomen off the floor. ○

23. He makes crawling movements when placed on his tummy – but does not move forward. ○

24. He can roll from his abdomen to his back. ○

25. He sits briefly without support. ○

26. He can take his weight on his feet if held upright. ○

27. When lying on his tummy he can take his weight on to his hands. ○

28. He bounces if held in an upright position. ○

29. When held upright he steps out to 'walk'. ○

30. While sitting he can adjust his posture when reaching. ○

31. He rocks on hands and knees and can make some forwards and/or backwards crawling movements. ○

32. He creeps around the room – but not necessarily by crawling. ○

33. He crawls. ○

34. He can adjust his posture when reaching forwards, but not always when reaching sideways. ○

35. He stands holding furniture. ○

36. He pulls himself up into a standing position. ○○○

37. He walks holding his parents' hands. ○○○

38. He can get himself from a lying to a sitting position. ○

39. He easily recovers his balance while sitting and reaching in any direction. ○

40. While standing, he lifts one foot to take a step. ○

41. He can reach for a toy that is behind him without toppling over. ○

42. He walks (cruises) around the furniture. ○

43. He stands with minimum support. ○

44. He reaches out to grab a toy or open a cupboard from a crawling position. ○

45. He walks holding your hand. ○

46. He cruises around furniture, and investigates what he finds, often letting go and standing without holding on. ○

47. He can get from a sitting to a standing position. ○

48. He crawls upstairs. ○

49. He takes a few steps without support. ○

50. He climbs onto the sofa, turns and sits. ○

51. He walks alone. ○

52. He crawls downstairs feet first. ○

53. He seats himself in a small chair. ○

54. He squats to pick up a small toy and returns to standing. ○

55. He pushes a toy truck in front of him when walking. ○

56. He pulls a toy on a string while walking.

57. He walks upstairs holding a parent's hand.

58. He bends from the waist to pick up toys without falling.

59. He walks backwards.

60. He walks downstairs holding a parent's hand.

61. He kicks a large stationary ball.

62. He climbs onto and off furniture.

63. He walks upstairs leading with one foot.

64. He walks downstairs leading with one foot.

65. He jumps off the bottom step of the stairs.

66. He jumps on the spot with both feet.

67. He alternates feet going upstairs.

68. He jumps off a low chair or from the bottom two steps of the stairs.

69. He walks on tiptoe.

70. He runs a short distance coordinating arm movements.

71. He uses his slide alone.

72. He pedals his trike.

73. He marches.

74. He stands on one foot.

75. He runs, changing direction without stopping.

76. He walks up and down stairs alternating feet.

77. He jumps forward 10 times without toppling over.

78. He jumps over a low hurdle.

79. He jumps backwards. ○

80. He hops on one foot. ○

81. He skips. ○

82. He walks backwards and forwards on a balance beam. ○

83. He can use a swing by himself. ○

84. He is able to play hopscotch. ○

85. He can skip with a rope that others turn. ○

KEY

The average baby will have completed the first 48 items in the first year, and item 81 by the time he is five years old. The breakdown is as follows:

1–4	month one	37–40	month 10
5–8	month two	41–44	month 11
9–12	month three	45–48	month 12
13–16	month four	49–58	year 1-2
17–20	month five	59–65	year 2-3
21–24	month six	66–74	year 3-4
25–28	month seven	75–81	year 4-5
29–32	month eight	82+	year five+
33–36	month nine		

The skilled movement and coordination checklist

Although skill development does not follow exactly the same pattern as mobility, it has many similarities. Because the motor control sequence starts at the head and moves down the body, and from the centre of the body outwards, the shoulders are controlled before the arms, the arms before the hands and the hands before the fingers. Although babies have little control over their fingers in the early months, they can manipulate objects using the innate clasping reflex. This is the grip a baby monkey uses to hold onto its mother. In the earliest days human babies close their hands over any object that touches the palm of their hand. This reflex can be easily tested by placing a finger in his hand – newborn babies grip so tightly that it is possible to pick them up while they hold tight to your fingers. In premature babies the toes grip equally hard and I am told that it is possible to hang a premature baby on a line by its fingers and toes – though I suspect this is something very few parents would consider trying!

The checklist opposite places the development of a child's motor skills more or less in order. Simply work through the questions one by one. The age at which the average child reaches these skilled movement milestones is given on page 47.

1. He has a strong grasp: you could lift him if he clutched your fingers. ○

2. His hands are usually closed. ○

3. He follows a slowly moving light (such as a small keyring torch) with his eyes. ○

4. His grasp is weakening. ○

5. His hands are beginning to open. ○

6. He turns his eyes to watch a moving finger. ○

7. He watches a toy dangled in front of him. ○

8. He will hold a rattle that is placed in his hand. ○

9. He hits dangling toys to make them move. ○

10. He reaches for toys placed in front of him but often overshoots. ○

11. He tries to grasp toys with both hands if they are offered to him. ○

12. He reaches and grasps using the palm of his hand and wrapping his fingers over the toy, but is unable to pick a toy up if he drops it. ○

13. He plays with his toes. ○

14. He picks up small objects between his fingers and thumb. ○

15. If you offer a second toy he drops the first. ○

16. He reaches for and picks up toys straight away. ○

17. He can hold one object while looking at another. ○

19. He picks things up and explores objects with his mouth. ○

19. He grasps his feet, pulling them to his mouth. ○

20. He holds his bottle (or your breast) when feeding. He holds the cup when you give him a drink. ○

21. He can transfer his toys from one hand to another. ○

22. He strokes a silky cloth or a carpet with a flat hand. ○

23. He bangs his spoon (or toys) on the table. ○

24. He pokes and prods with a finger. ○

25. He rakes toys towards him. ○

26. He releases and drops toys by letting them roll off his open hand. ○

27. He opposes his thumb with the tip of his index finger (a pincer grip) to pick up small items like peas. ○

28. He can hold two toys while looking at a third. ○

29. He can squeeze a squeaky toy. ○

30. He releases and drops objects by turning his hand over and opening his fingers. ○

31. He claps. ○

32. He bangs the table with his hand. ○

33. He scoops up food or sand with a spoon. ○

34. He has a dominant hand. ○

35. He can put small objects into a container. ○

36. He can imitate drinking when given a cup. ○

37. He can imitate hair brushing. ○

38. He can feed himself with a spoon – even if messily. ○

39. He can pick up a beaker and drink.

40. He can hand things to people, letting them go.

41. He will imitate if you roll a ball to him.

42. He can put four rings on a peg.

43. He can take a peg out of a peg board – or take apart a simple construction toy.

44. He can put the simplest shapes (circle, triangle) in his shape sorter.

45. He can build a tower of three bricks.

46. He is able to make a mark with a crayon.

47. He tries to brush his teeth.

48. He can string four large beads.

49. He can turn doorknobs.

50. He can throw a beanbag or a small ball.

51. He can throw a ball to someone standing a metre and a half away.

52. He can turn the pages of a book.

53. He is able to unwrap a small present.

54. He can build a tower of five bricks.

55. He can fold a piece of paper in half.

56. He is able to take apart and put together a construction of large interlacing bricks such as Lego.

57. He can unscrew a nesting toy.

58. He can roll a ball of play dough.

59. He can use a rolling pin. ○

60. He is able to put three pieces into a form board puzzle. ○

61. He can snip a narrow paper strip with blunt scissors. ○

62. He can catch a large ball if you throw it into his arms. ○

63. He can trace around a template. ○

64. He puts on most of his clothes without asking for help. ○

65. He can wash and dry his hands. ○

66. He is able to twist and untwist a screw cap bottle lid. ○

67. He can bounce and catch a large ball. ○

68. He is able to make and cut shapes with play dough. ○

69. He draws rudimentary figures. ○

70. He can cut along a curved line. ○

71. He can colour in without going over too many edges. ○

72. He draws simple, recognisable pictures – houses, animals, people, cars, buses. ○

73. He can put together simple construction kits. ○

74. He can cut around a circle. ○

75. He can cut and paste simple shapes. ○

76. He can colour in with less than 10% going outside the line. ○

77. He can print a few capital letters. ○

78. He can touch his thumb to each finger. ○

79. He can copy a few lower case letters. ○

80. He can hit a nail with a hammer. ○

KEY

The average baby will have completed the first 36 items in the first year, and item 70 by the time he is five years old. The breakdown is as follows:

1–3	month one	28–30	month 10
4–6	month two	31–33	month 11
7–9	month three	34–36	month 12
10–12	month four	37–41	months 12–18
13–15	month five	42–47	months 19–24
16–18	month six	48–60	year 2-3
19–21	month seven	61–66	year 3-4
22–24	month eight	67–70	year 4-5
25–27	month nine	70 +	year five+

Top Tips

1. Always encourage your child to believe 'I can do it.'

2. Build up his self-esteem with praise and with frequently expressed love and admiration.

3. Expect him to try.

4. Let him try – do not rush in to help too soon.

5. Talk to him face-to-face – getting down to his level.

6. Show him how and set a good example – children learn by imitating what we do.

7. Minimise criticism. He should always be praised more often than he is criticised.

8. Do not stereotype. A child who thinks he is badly behaved often fulfils the prophecy.

9. A novel toy or game attracts, but to sustain interest it should be appropriate for his age. Read the labels on toy boxes and make toys appropriate to his age and stage.

10. Put away toys he is not using: a toy that is around and not played with is unlikely to sustain his interest.

Chapter 2

Children's Cognitive Skills: Thinking, Learning and Remembering

In this chapter we examine the way children think and how their memories develop: skills that psychologists and teachers often group together as cognition. The first section includes a group of general tests of various cognitive abilities arranged by age. These should show you the child's developmental stage. They are followed by a group of developmental checklists showing you the things toddlers can do at various ages, and a checklist that shows the characteristics one might find in a talented child. The final section includes some classic experiments that give you a little window into your child's way of thinking.

 ## Learning in the First Months

The major challenge for the newborn is to come to know the world around her. Viewed with the experience of many years, it is hard to imagine that at birth she does not know where her body stops and the rest of the world begins. She does not yet know which things move of their own accord (animals) and which move as a result of external forces. Nor does she understand object identity – she thinks, for example, that you are a new Mother every time she sees you. Nor does she understand object permanence – that things continue to exist even when she cannot see them. In their first months children must also learn that actions have specific consequences, that objects exist in a spatial framework, and that the same object may look quite different when approached from another angle.

HOW EXACTLY DO BABIES GO ABOUT LEARNING?

Most psychologists today believe that both nature and nurture inter-act continuously to guide development. We know that virtually all children go through the same sequence of motor development (suggesting the unfolding of an innate programme) but, within limits, practice accelerates process and lack of 'normal' experience slows development. For example, almost all children learn to speak – but not before they have reached a certain level of neurological development. However much you shape a child's language they will not learn to put words together to form sentences until the second year of life. Equally if you do not shape their language they will start putting together sentences much later than this – but providing they are exposed to language they will manage to do so. In most instances practice affects the rate at which a skill develops, but unless experience is outside the normal range it does not influence the ultimate level of skill. Clearly this does not apply to the acquisition of what we might loosely call culturally transmitted knowledge – history, mathematics, music, art, sport, athletics – which are, as we are all aware, much more dependent on innate ability and practice.

NOT QUITE LIKE US

Babies live in the here and now, supplemented by whatever memories are cued by what they currently see, hear and smell. As they sit in their pushchairs they see what they see in the moment, and feel the emotions they feel in the moment and the only things they add to that experience are those that are cued by the present circumstances. In essence they can think: 'When I last had this coat on I went for a walk' or 'When I last smelt that smell Mummy changed my nappy' but not 'I had spaghetti for dinner yesterday' or 'Daddy went to work early today' because sitting in their pushchair there is nothing to remind them of spaghetti or Daddy. Nor do any of the things they remember have the clarity and order that words give them and, without this, babies have difficulty consciously organising and integrating separately stored episodic memories (things that happened in different times and different places) into 'theories' and 'ideas' of how things work. They learn by experience but only if the memory of that experience is cued by their current context. They do not integrate knowledge acquired at different times and in different contexts to form a reasoned view of how the world works – as older children and adult humans do. The tests below help us to see our child's progression from a baby's way of thinking towards something more akin to our own.

The following tests examine your child's cognitive skills. There are separate tests for:

❑ 6–12 months
❑ 1–2 years
❑ 2–3 years
❑ 3–4 years
❑ 4–5 years

Select the test appropriate to the child's age. If your child is close to the age boundary you may want to do the test above and below her age range.

SCORING THE TESTS

Your child gets a score of 1 for everything she can do. So, for example, she would get 1 if she can do the item listed under 'a', an extra 1 if she can also do 'b', and another if she can do 'c':

❑ a alone scores 1, a+b scores 2, a+b+c scores 3.

Thinking, Learning and Memory: 6–12 Months

1. Does your child

a) Become excited when she makes something happen, such as knocking a toy and making it move? ○

b) Anticipate the 'And down into the ditch' when you play 'This is the way the ladies ride'? ○

c) Know what comes next in her book? ○

2. Does your child

a) Anticipate she is about to be fed? ○

b) Recognise a toy she has not seen for a couple of weeks? ○

c) Remember the faces of adults she does not see very often? ○

3. Does your child

a) Imitate actions such as poking out her tongue or opening and closing her mouth? ○

b) Imitate actions such as waving bye-bye? ○

c) Pretend to feed a doll or drink from a toy cup? ○

4. Does your child

a) Watch her hands? ○

b) Look from one object to another as if comparing them? ○

c) Look for an object that has rolled out of sight? ○

5. Can your child

a) Play peek-a-boo?

b) Remove a toy from a container?

c) Push three blocks train-style?

6. Does your child

a) Look at multiple reflections of her mother in two dressing table mirrors with delight?

b) Cry or avoid looking at multiple reflections of her mother in two dressing table mirrors?

c) When looking at her reflection pat and talk to the baby in the mirror?

7. Does your child

a) Reach for toys on the left and right?

b) Look for a toy that is partly hidden under a cloth?

c) Look for a toy that is completely hidden under a cloth?

9. Does your child

a) Bang toys or explore them with her mouth?

b) Play with each toy in a different but appropriate manner?

c) Look up from her game – and then go back to it?

9. Does your child

a) Know family members by the sound of their voices? ○
b) Show her pleasure at seeing you? ○
c) Call out to you when you come into the room? ○

10. Does your child

a) Recognise her name? ○
b) Understand the meaning of 'no'? ○
c) Know the names of two or more body parts (but cannot
   say them)? ○

INTERPRETING THE SCORES

❑ The average six-month-old may not be able to do everything on
   the 'a' list, but should be able to get an 'a' for the majority of
   questions. *Expected score about 8–9.*

❑ The average nine-month-old should get most of the 'a's with
   some 'b's. *Expected score of 13–15.*

❑ The average 12-month-old should get most of the 'b's and a few
   'c's. *Expected score of 24–26.*

Thinking, Learning and Memory: 1–2 Years

1. Can your child

a) Find a toy you hide under a cloth? ○

b) Take six bricks out of a container one by one? ○

c) Place a toy in a box, on a chair and under a cloth when asked? ○

2. Can your child

a) Point to one body part such as her nose? ○

b) Point to five different body parts? ○

c) Point to 10 parts of her body? ○

3. Can your child

a) Place one round shape in her shape sorter or put a peg figure into a toy car? ○

b) Stack three bricks one on top of the other? ○

c) Place five or more rings on a stacking toy in the right order? ○

4. If you show your child a Lego brick of a certain size and colour can she

a) Transfer it to one hand while she picks up another brick with the other hand? ○

b) Find another just like it? ○

c) If you start with three different bricks can she find a brick to match each one? ○

5. If you encourage your child will she

a) Copy you when you bang on the table? ○

b) Imitate you when you pretend to rock her doll to sleep? ○

c) Imitate a simple sequence of actions such as washing toy dishes and putting them to drain? ○

6. Will your child

a) Push along a small car or toy train? ○

b) Push along a toy car or train (or sit in a pedal car) making noises such as 'Brmmm' or 'Toot-toot'? ○

c) Pretend a box is a toy car – including making noises or pretending to steer? ○

7. If you show your child a book will she

a) Enjoy turning the pages? ○

b) Recognise a few pictures? ○

c) Listen to a simple story? ○

8. Can your child

a) Hold a crayon? ○

b) Scribble? ○

c) Copy a vertical line you draw? ○

9. When looking at a book together does your child

a) Look where you look and point? ○

b) Point to a picture of a cat when you ask her where the cat is? ○

c) Find the cat in a later picture by turning pages? ○

10. Does your child

a) Know her name? ○

b) Point to herself when asked by name, e.g. 'Where is Amy?' ○

c) Point to herself when asked 'Where is my very best girl?' ○

INTERPRETING THE SCORES

❑ The average one-year-old may not be able to do everything on the 'a' list, but should be able to get an 'a' for the majority of questions. *Expected score about 8–9.*

❑ The average 18-month-old should get most of the 'a's with some 'b's. *Expected score of 13–5.*

❑ The average two-year-old should get most of the 'b's and a few 'c's. *Expected score of 24–26.*

Thinking, Learning and Memory: 2–3 Years

1. Does your child

a) Know the name of some of the numbers under 10 but not the order?

b) Know at least some of the sequence of numbers 1–10 (such as one-two-three or five-six-seven) but does not get the entire sequence right every time and is very uncertain after 10?

c) Know the sequence of numbers 1–10 and the name of some higher numbers – although not necessarily the order of these numbers?

2. If your child is playing can she

a) Look up and answer a question and then go back to her game?

b) Fetch something she needs from across the room and then go back to her game?

c) Go into another room to find something she needs and then go back to her game?

3. Can your child

a) Carry out simple pretend actions such as rocking a baby doll?

b) Play simple domestic pretend games (such as cooking in the kitchen) with other children? ○

c) Organise other children to play such games? ○

4. Does your child

a) Enjoy dressing up but wears the clothes, rather than pretending to be the person? ○

b) Dress up but not always play the part she is dressed to play? ○

c) Put on the clothes that mark the role – especially when playing with others? ○

5. Can your child

a) Turn the pages in a book to find a particular picture? ○

b) Find the book you ask her to find? ○

c) Tell you what happens next in a simple story? ○

6. If you ask your child will she be able to

a) Stack three blocks one on top of the other? ○

b) Put three different-shaped pieces into a tray puzzle? ○

c) Stack five or more rings on a peg in the correct order (i.e. large at the bottom, small at the top)? ○

7. Can your child

a) Match a toy to a picture of that toy? ○

b) Put together pairs of socks or shoes? ○

c) Say whether two things are the same or different? ○

8. If you put a smudge of lipstick on your child's forehead and then sit with her looking in the mirror does she

a) Look at the mark in the mirror and maybe even try to rub it off the child in the mirror? ○

b) Rub her own forehead? ○

c) Comment on the fact that she has a mark on her forehead? ○

9. Can your child

a) Name pictures? ○

b) Name actions? ○

c) Name at least three colours? ○

10. Can your child

a) Name the animal that makes a certain sound? ○

b) Name objects that make a certain sound? ○

c) Carry out the actions for an action rhyme? ○

INTERPRETING THE SCORES

❑ The average two-year-old may not be able to do everything on the 'a' list, but should be able to get an 'a' for the majority of questions. *Expected score about 8–9.*

❏ The average two-and-a-half-year-old should get most of the 'a's with some 'b's. *Expected score of 13–15.*

❏ The average three-year-old should get most of the 'a's and 'b's and a few 'c's. *Expected score of 24–26.*

Thinking, Learning and Memory: 3–4 Years

1. Can your child

a) Point to five body parts when asked? ○

b) Point to 10 body parts when asked? ○

c) Point to a missing part of a picture when asked? ○

2. Can your child

a) Pick out two things that are the same colour? ○

b) Name three colours? ○

c) Name eight colours? ○

3. Can your child draw a man with

a) Limbs added to a body that you have drawn? ○

b) Head, body and all four limbs? ○

c) Head, body, four limbs and details such as fingers? ○

4. Is your child able to count

a) Up to three? ○

b) Up to 10? ○

c) Up to 20? ○

5. Can your child

a) Copy when you draw a cross and a circle? ○

b) Copy when you draw a V? ○

c) Copy when you draw a group of Vs, VVVVVVV? ○

6. Can your child tell you

a) If a toy is big or little? ○

b) If a vegetable is heavy or light? ○

c) What times of day are associated with different activities? ○

7. Can your child

a) Arrange objects (such as spoons and forks) into categories? ○

b) Tell you which objects (knife and fork, egg and eggcup) go together? ○

c) Lay the table with cutlery, glasses, table napkins, etc? ○

9. Can your child

a) Put three different shapes in her shape sorter? ○

b) Build a bridge with three bricks? ○

c) Complete a six-piece puzzle? ○

9. Can your child

a) Find a particular book (or DVD) when you ask her to? ○

b) Say which object has been removed from a group of three? ○

c) Recall four animals seen in a picture? ○

10. If asked can your child

a) Name three actions? ○

b) Name three colours? ○

c) Name three shapes? ○

INTERPRETING THE SCORES

❑ The average three-year-old may not be able to do everything on the 'a' list, but should be able to get an 'a' for the majority of questions. *Expected score about 8–9.*

❑ The average three-and-a-half-year-old should get most of the 'a's with some 'b's. *Expected score of 13–15.*

❑ The average four-year-old should get most of the 'b's and a few 'c's. *Expected score of 24–26.*

Thinking, Learning and Memory: 4–5 Years

1. If you put three cars in a row, can your child

a) Identify the first or last? ○

b) Identify the first and last? ○

c) Identify the first, middle and last? ○

2. Can your child

a) Say what happens next in a simple repetitive story? ○

b) Tell you five main facts from a story read three times? ○

c) Sing five lines of a song? ○

3. When your child writes her name on her drawings, or copies something you have drawn for her, does she place it neatly on the page or run out of space?

a) She often runs out of space. ○

b) She can place things neatly if reminded. ○

c) She plans how things fit onto the page although she may need prompting. ○

4. Do your child's drawings of people have

a) Heads, faces and maybe arms? ○

b) Heads, faces, bodies and arms or legs? ○

c) Heads, faces, bodies, arms, legs and details such as fingers or knees? ○

5. Does your child follow instructions?

a) Sometimes. ○

b) Usually, providing they are not too complex. ○

c) Always, unless she chooses not to. ○

6. If your child tries to make a construction from boxes

a) Does she fail to plan? ○

b) Does she make some plans? ○

c) Is she self-critical? ○

7. If you are sitting with your back to the window, would your child

a) Talk about things you cannot see without understanding
   you did not see what she did? ○

b) Talk about what you can both see? ○

c) Explain what you could not see? ○

8. If you ask your child to pick an ending to jokes such as 'Why is the sand wet' would she

a) Pick an answer at random? ○

b) Pick the truthful answer, 'Because the wave splashed'? ○

c) Pick the joke, 'Because the sea weed'? ○

9. Can your child

a) Look up from what she is doing and then go back to
   that task? ○

b) Talk to others as she plays? ○

c) Break off from doing something and return sometime later? ○

10. When your child has been somewhere without you does she

a) Tell you about it as if you had been there ('He hit me')? ⠀⠀⠀○

b) Explain some things but not enough for you to completely follow ('Tom hit me on the slide')? ⠀⠀⠀○

c) Explain the background so you can understand ('Tom is a boy at my school, he bumped into me on the slide')? ⠀⠀⠀○

INTERPRETING THE SCORES

❏ The average four-year-old may not be able to do everything on the 'a' list, but should be able to get an 'a' for the majority of questions. *Expected score about 8–9.*

❏ The average four-and-a-half-year-old should get most of the 'a's with some 'b's. *Expected score of 13–15.*

❏ The average five-year-old should get most of the 'b's and a few 'c's. *Expected score of 24–26.*

The Learning Checklists

The following checklists outline 10 things most children can do and understand by the time they are a certain age.

By the time she is two-and-a-half

1. She can identify her family and friends in photographs. ⠀⠀⠀○

2. She can investigate why things happen. She might, for example, hide a little car behind the door of her toy garage – and then open the door, take out the car and do it again. Or she might blow bubbles in her milk with a straw, watch the bubbles subside and then do it again. ○

3. She watches and becomes engrossed in activities. She might, for example, pour water from a jug into her bath, watching the water carefully as it leaves the jug and flows into the bath. ○

4. She can identify herself in photographs. ○

5. She recognises herself in the mirror – if you put a mark on her head that she sees for the first time when she looks in the mirror, she reaches to her head (not the mirror head) to rub it off. ○

6. She plays pretend games with other children – these do not have a complex story line but rather centre on shared experiences: domestic tasks, shopping, driving. ○

7. She ascribes human properties to animals and objects. ○

8. She knows if you turn over two pages in her favourite book. ○

9. She can remember simple songs and rhymes – especially those with actions. ○

10. She can sort toys into simple categories – such as toy cars and toy bricks. ○

By the time she is three

1. She is able to gossip and pass the time of day with other children and with adults. ○

2. She can tell simple factual stories – and may do so during play. ○

3. She can remember what happened yesterday. ○

4. She can remember exciting events – such as a trip to the zoo – from the more distant past. ○

5. Situations elicit memories – she remembers what she saw in the park the last time she visited, but may not have mentioned this before. Such memories may be for events that occurred weeks and months previously. ○

6. She occasionally repeats things to help her to remember – but does not do so systematically. ○

7. She can arrange things into simple categories – such as toy cars and toy tractors or pictures of birds and pictures of airplanes. ○

8. She can compare things by size saying which is the biggest and which is the smallest and may be able to do this for high and low and long and short – but not reliably. ○

9. She can complete a three- to four-piece jigsaw and put together a four-piece nesting toy. ○

10. She can draw a horizontal and a vertical line, but has problems drawing a diagonal line, so she can draw a cross, but finds a V shape difficult.

By the time she is three-and-a-half

1. She still talks as if you share her experience and sees what you see.

2. She can do jigsaws and puzzles of four or more pieces and put together two parts of a shape to make a whole. (For example, if you cut a circle or a picture of a car in two.)

3. She can sort things into categories on the basis of one attribute (for example, sort the whites from coloured washing, or her clothes from your clothes, but not both – her white clothes from your white clothes).

4. She can match things one to one (putting a cup on each saucer, giving each teddy a plate).

5. She draws enclosed spaces – circles, squares and lines and crosses. She still scribbles but her pictures are balanced rather than irregularly placed on the page.

6. Her understanding of causality (what makes something happen) depends on how close things are, for example, she may think that the engine noise makes the car go.

7. She believes death is transient.

8. She may believe bad things happen because she is naughty. ○

9. She thinks if A causes B, then B causes A. So if she bumped into the chair, the chair bumped into her. ○

10. She knows whether she is a girl (or he is a boy) but not that she has always been that gender and always will be. ○

By the time she is four

1. She can gossip and talk about the past and the future. ○

2. She can explain why she thinks something happened. ○

3. She draws people with irregularly shaped heads, eyes are often placed near the edge of the head or together on the left-hand side of the face. ○

4. She can add legs to an incomplete man. ○

5. She enjoys constructing things but does not always plan ahead, so towers topple and things do not fit together. She gets very frustrated when this happens. ○

6. Her movements are smooth and efficient, she eats and drinks without dropping food. ○

7. She lines up jigsaw pieces before trying to put them in and may be able to connect a piece to two or three other pieces at the same time. ○

8. She can copy a bridge you have built and copy a sequence or pattern of bricks or beads. ○

9. She is able to dress herself although she still makes mistakes – such as getting her shoes on the wrong feet or her pants on the wrong way around. ○

10. She can put together simple toy kits, draw a square and name three shapes such as triangle, circle and square. ○

By the time she is four-and-a-half

1. She can take the perspective of another child and relate this to her own. For example, when talking to someone she is facing about what she can see through the window she will explain that it is behind the listener. ○

2. She realises that your thoughts and feelings are separate from hers and takes this into account when she reports what she did at nursery or preschool. ○

3. She draws human figures with faces, eyes and noses. They may have legs but probably not bodies. ○

4. She draws simple houses and buildings and may begin to draw crude boats and cars. ○

5. She can name the time of day that is associated with various activities (breakfast, school, bedtime). ○

6. She can put together two or more ideas and form a conclusion. ○

7. She can set the table and sort things into different groups. ○

9. She may be able to recognise letters and numbers and, if encouraged, may be able to write her name. ○

9. She can wash her face and clean her teeth, and dress herself in all but the most difficult items. ○

10. She can repeat a simple rhyme and carry out all the actions. ○

By the time she is five

1. She can play simple board games but does not use strategy. ○

2. She remembers where she left things and does well in games that challenge this ability. ○

3. She can count and understands that three is more than two, but may not understand that seven is more than six. ○

4. She dresses herself, puts on her coat and shoes but still needs help with laces, zips and gloves. ○

5. She eats neatly and is able to use a knife and fork but still needs help cutting up meat. ○

6. She coordinates two or more ideas to form a conclusion, or puts together a short sequence of actions in a skilled way. ○

7. She tells jokes but does not understand why they are funny. ○

9. She can add legs and arms to her drawings and draws houses and cars. ○

9. She is beginning to plan ahead and follow simple

instructions so she can make more complex constructions and deal with kits with smaller pieces.

10. She can colour in outline drawings and form most of her letters, she can wash her face, brush her teeth and dry her hands and face – but does not dry her body.

Is She Talented?

It is impossible to say exactly where talent comes from. We suspect that genes are involved, and we know upbringing and training are important. But if the right genes and the right training were enough, talented individuals would never arrive on the scene as if from nowhere: and, of course, they often do. Outstanding talent is more than the sum of the skills. There are many people who have good voices or draw well – but the really talented are able to capture emotion in their voices and paint pictures that speak to us and move us – and quite where that ability comes from nobody really knows.

The talent test: spotting a talent for art, music and drama

SCORING THE TEST

For each question below assign a value between 0 and 3.

❏ 0 means no, this isn't really true

❏ 1 means yes, this is true

☐ 2 means yes, this is very true
☐ 3 means yes, this is exceptionally true

1. Have her drawings always been balanced? When she started to scribble was the scribble well placed on the page with as much to the right as to the left? ○

2. Has she always drawn without encouragement? ○

3. Was she quick to manage fiddly things like doing up coat buttons? ○

4. Compared with her peers do her drawings and paintings have more detail? Could she draw a face before she was three? At five do her pictures tell a story? Can she convey movement? ○

5. Does she turn to drawing to sooth and calm herself? Does she express emotions in what she draws? For example, do her drawings look different when she is angry from when she is happy? ○

6. Does she experiment with colour and composition? Has she started to vary the orientation of her figures or do all her animals and people still stare directly out of the page? ○

7. Does she draw both happy and sad faces? Does she draw what she sees rather than what should be there? ○

8. Does she prefer stories to factual books? ○

9. By the age of three did a story sooth her when she was feeling sad? ○

10. At four could she make up stories? ○

11. Does she tell tall tales? ○

12. Can she play without someone organising the activity? ○

13. Does she mix pretence with more physical activities like bike riding? ○

14. Is she better than most at imitating sounds and actions? ○

15. Does your child move with more grace than other children of her age? ○

16. Is she agile? Does she enjoy physical activity? ○

17. Does musical ability and appreciation run in your family? ○

18. Has she always responded to music? Does it sooth her when she is sad? ○

19. Does she sing and dance when she is happy? Does she have a natural sense of rhythm? At three could she clap and move to music? ○

20. Can she sing better than most of her peers? ○

21. Does she join in when others sing or play music? ○

INTERPRETING THE SCORES

Add up the scores for each section.

❑ Qs 1–7 relate to art   Score.......

❑ Qs 8–14 to drama   Score.......

❑ Qs 15–21 to music   Score.......

The higher the score, the more likely your child is to have a special talent. Note, however, that some questions are age-dependent. It is highly unlikely that any child under three would get a score as high as 21 (the maximum score) in any section. A talented 4–5-year-old might get a score close to this.

THE UP-SIDE: FOSTERING TALENT

Parents can and do influence the talents of their children whether directly, by teaching and guiding their learning, or indirectly by believing in their child's capabilities and persuading the child to share that belief. Few parents question that this is good parenting. Long-term follow-up studies of early intervention programmes, such as Head Start in the USA that educated and stretched preschoolers from poor and deprived homes, show that those who attended such programmes in the 1980s are more likely to be leading successful lives today. Few question that providing education for children, and parental involvement in that education, is good and that includes fostering special talents.

THE DOWN-SIDE: HOTHOUSING CHILDREN

It may seem straightforward to assume that if a little help is good for children, isn't a lot even better? Investigations into child protégées suggest that most child 'geniuses' have in the background an ambitious parent who organises their talent with a firm hand. It has been identified that some parents of talented children often devote their lives to their child's 'genius'.

If this was the only way for children to succeed we might not question it. But it is not. Tennis and golf excepted, the majority of those who excel in their field did not excel as children. Early and zealous teaching programmes do not suit all children, and they frequently do not suit all parent–child relationships. There are talented children who fail to reach their parents' high standards and who sometimes suffer 'baby burn out' as a consequence. Other children can simply stop progressing any further because of their fear of failing. When musicologists examine the skills of those who began piano lessons early, and continued to play, and those who started early but stopped there was no difference in their underlying musical abilities – or in their love for music. Some just opted out. Interestingly those who started music lessons later (at about the age of eight) were less likely to give up. Some who succeed as children fail to make the transition into adult success, perhaps because the motivation was never their own. The role of parent 'fanclub' to a child's success is never an attractive one – and all too frequently there is a breakdown in the relationship between a driving parent and the child star.

 ## Learning About the World

In this section we examine some classic experiments that tell us something of the way in which the child views the world. They help remind us that children are not just little people: they are people who think and remember things in a different way from us. Children are not just smaller than adults, they are physically and mentally immature by comparison. A child's body is not just a smaller version of an adult body, it is a different shape; and a child's hand is not just smaller, it is also much less skilled.

The brain is like the body and the hand: both smaller in childhood and more immature. At birth the brain is only a third the size of the adult brain, and there are still many connections to be formed. Not only do children know less than their parents, they also think differently. In this section we will look at some of those thinking patterns. Let us start with a little test for you to do:

1. What month comes after July?
2. What is the capital of France?
3. What is your mother's first name?
4. What is 8+6?
5. Where did you spend Christmas last year?
6. How are the three dots arranged on a dice?
7. How are the three hearts arranged on a playing card?
8. What are the letters on the bottom line of a typewriter?
9. What does freshly baked bread smell like?
10. What does chocolate taste like?

Most of us will have immediate answers to the first five questions, but we have to stop and think about the dice, playing card and typewriter, and may not be able to answer the last two questions even though we know that most of us would immediately recognise the smell of freshly baked bread and the taste of chocolate. This is not because tastes and smells are any less familiar – we have probably eaten chocolate more recently than we have watched the roll of a dice. We have difficulties when we cannot easily put things into words: there is no question that language changes the way we think and the way we remember what we think.

In their first year, young children do not have language to support thought or help memory and even after they can speak they do not automatically put those things they need to remember into words. This means that the way they think about things is often quite different from the way adults think and different from the way they will think and remember once they grow up.

Learning about objects

If you photograph a cup from above it is a very different shape than it would be if photographed from the side. If viewed from 60 centimetres the photograph shows a much bigger cup than if the picture were taken from a distance of three metres. Because we move around our environment, the 'images' of the objects that fall on the retina of our eye and are analysed by our brains are constantly changing although the objects themselves remain the same. Testing to see whether babies have developed constancy (the technical name for understanding that a cup is still a cup whatever our angle of view) is too complex to easily do at home: but there are other aspects of objects that babies learn about in the first year and these are much easier to test. We will look at two: identity (that this is the same object I saw a moment ago) and permanence (that this object will continue to exist even if I stop looking at it).

WHAT BABIES HAVE TO LEARN ABOUT OBJECTS

Object constancy Knowing that an object viewed from different angles and in different lights remains the same. By 4–5 months children show evidence that they have learned about object constancy.

Object identity Knowing that this object is the one that they saw last time. Children show evidence of this by 5–6 months.

Object permanence Knowing that objects continue to exist even when they can no longer be seen. Children begin to show evidence of this at about seven months, but do not fully understand until they are 10–14 months.

TESTING FOR OBJECT IDENTITY

This is a simple experiment to see whether your baby realises she only has one mother. Child psychologists have used this test to examine how soon the child knows there should only be one mother. They found that younger babies were delighted to see lots of mothers and lots of babies – but that some time around the age of 5–6 months children stopped liking all those mothers. They knew there should only be one – so when they saw mothers stretching away into the distance some cried, some looked away and some others looked puzzled. This is the reaction you are looking for. When it happens you know your child understands object identity.

You will need
❑ A table with angled mirrors arranged to show lots of repeated images.
❑ A chair to sit in front of the mirror with your baby on your lap.

What to do
Arrange the mirrors so they give only one view. Sit in front of the mirror with your baby on your lap facing the mirrors. Point to your reflection. At this age she will not recognise herself, but will recognise your reflection. Now rearrange the mirrors so there are lots of babies and lots of mums. How does she react?

TESTING FOR OBJECT PERMANENCE
Child psychologists have used this test to examine the development of the child's understanding that objects continue to exist even when she cannot see them. At 5–7 months you will almost certainly find that

your child loses interest in the toy if she cannot see it; but by 8–12 months she will begin to search for the toy hidden under the cloth. Initially she will only do so if more than half of the toy is showing – but gradually will look even when only a bit of the toy is showing. Eventually she will look even when the toy is completely hidden. Object permanence develops over a number of months. Here are some simple experiments to check the stage your child has reached.

You will need

❑ Two contrasting toys – say a teddy and a toy train.

❑ A cloth to cover the toys and a piece of card big enough to hide the toys behind.

❑ A table and a chair for the child to sit on.

What to do

Sit the baby at the table and give her the teddy to play with. After a minute or two distract her for a moment while you take away the toy, place it on the table and completely cover it with the cloth. Watch what the child does. If she ignores the toy, take it from under the cloth and then repeat the test but this time only half cover the toy.

Other things to try

❑ Hide the teddy under the cloth 10 times and let your baby find the teddy. Now take a second cloth and this time show the child you are hiding the teddy under this new cloth. You will almost certainly find that the child looks for the teddy under the cloth where she usually finds it.

❏ Instead of a teddy use a small finger puppet or similar-sized doll. Show the child that you have hidden the doll in the usual way – but remove the doll as you put the cloth over. Now remove the cloth. Even children as young as five months will look surprised when they do not see anything under the cloth.

❏ Do the test again but this time add a second doll rather than removing the first one. Remove the cloth. Children as young as five months may look surprised when they see the extra doll.

❏ After showing her that you have put the doll under the cloth remove the doll and replace it with something very different. Children who were surprised to find nothing under the cloth may show no sign of surprise when they find something they have not seen before under the cloth. At first, children know there should be one object – but not what that object is.

TESTING HOW LONG YOUR BABY CAN REMEMBER

This is a simple experiment to see how long your baby remembers. Child psychologists have used this test to examine the development of memory. They found that two-month-old babies who had learned to make the pompoms move started to kick immediately they were placed under the pompoms the next day; but did not remember what to do if the delay between pompom sessions was more than three days. By three months they would kick immediately if the gap between the sessions was a week – but not if it was two weeks. By six months they remembered at two weeks but not three. Over the next months there is a steady progression, with babies remembering what to do for longer periods between the sessions.

You will need

- [ ] A piece of thick rope or elastic to tie across the cot or playpen, or alternatively use a play mat with a flexible plastic arch. (The arch should move when the ribbon attached to the arch is pulled – see below.)
- [ ] Five pompoms (or use Christmas tree baubles, but not glass ones or any with sharp corners) or coloured cards, to tie on the rope.
- [ ] A ribbon loosely attached to the child's ankle so that when the baby kicks she makes the arch shake and as a consequence the pompoms move.

What to do

Hang the pompoms from the rope or plastic arch and loosely attach the arch to the baby's foot with a ribbon. Now when the baby kicks she makes the arch move and this makes the pompoms jiggle – and all you have to watch is how long your baby takes to discover this. Once she is beginning to tire of the task take the pompoms away.

Then try again sometime later. How quickly does the child start to kick second time around? Is it faster than first time around?

Other things to try

❑ **Can small babies count?** Try the above experiment with four pompoms and, before giving the second test, either add another pompom or take one away. Does this make a difference? If your baby kicks for longer the second time, she must remember enough about the first display to realise that things have changed.

❑ **Has she really forgotten?** If you give your baby a few reminders (put her under the pompoms without attaching the ribbon) on the day before you do the second pompom test you may find she remembers to kick when she sees the pompoms. Some children remember (after the reminder) for up to a month – even at an age when they would not normally remember for more than a few days.

WHEN CAN YOUR BABY FORM CATEGORIES?

In order to be able to understand what words mean, babies must be able to form categories: to be able to divide the world up into plants and animals, tables and chairs or cats and dogs. They must learn to make the groupings to which they eventually attach words.

One way of testing whether or not babies are able to form categories before they start to speak is to show them a series of items that are all in the *same* category along with *one* item which is from another category – and see whether the baby looks at the 'out of category' picture more intently or for longer than she looks at 'in category' examples. If she does, she must be able to form the category. So, for example, you might show her six pairs of cat pictures. In each pair the cats are in different positions, are different breeds or have different coat colours. If the child recognises that these are all members of one category – cats – she will show more interest in a picture (say of a dog or a pig), which belongs to a different category.

Child psychologists have used this test to examine the development of concepts. By 3–4 months children look longer at the 'out of category' item (in this case the dog), demonstrating that by this age they are able to form the category 'cat'. The test can be repeated to show that the child is able to make other animal categories (horses, pigs) as well as categories such as cars, tractors, houses, etc. They can also make larger overriding categories such as animal or buildings. (In this case the first pairs are different sorts of animals, and the last one an animal and a house – or vice versa.)

You will need

❑ Seven pictures of animals or objects that belong to the same category. You could choose seven pictures of different breeds of cat or seven different makes of car.

❑ One 'out of category' picture. In the case of the cat picture the other might be a dog. In the case of cars it could be a lorry.

What to do

Arrange the cat pictures in contrasting pairs so the two cats that form the pair are different breeds, have different coats and are in different positions each time. The final pair is a picture of a cat and a picture of a dog.

Show the child the six cat pictures. Then show her the picture of the cat and the dog. When she looks at the final pair does she show more interest in the dog than the cat?

Top Tips

1. Help her to concentrate: keep toys that are out of use out of sight.

2. Remove distractions: keep noise to a minimum when she needs to concentrate and turn off the TV. Children find it hard to look away from visual stimulation.

3. Children find it easier to concentrate if they are not restless. Encourage her to let off steam before settling down to work. Let her race around to music or jump off the settee onto a pile of cushions.

4. If you need to tell her something important get down to her level and talk face-to-face.

5. Discuss things, answer her questions and encourage her to ask them.

6. Children find it easier to remember if they have cues to remind them. A regular routine will help them progress from day to day.

7. Expect competence and praise achievement.

8. Allow mess. Children cannot learn if they are afraid of getting their clothes dirty or dripping water or paint.

9. Tell her how clever she is.

10. Remember a toy or game that is too advanced for her does not advance her knowledge or her competence. Instead it frustrates progress.

Chapter 3
The Language Tests

Even though they all do it, and their chatter becomes commonplace before long, a baby's first words are a small miracle – and one that is followed by many other small miracles as language emerges and matures. There is an old saying that the eyes are the 'window to the soul', but for small children language surely plays that role. It is the things they say that open their minds to us. 'Is this another sort of paradise?' my young son asked as we walked into the wood one misty autumn morning. Suddenly the bustle and noise of London stopped and I looked at it through his eyes. He was right. Even today if I cut through the wood on winter mornings and see the light coming sideways through the trees as he did then, I remember his words. Most parents will at some time be floored by the things their children say; from such little things comes happiness.

Language springs from a child's desire to engage the social world. Although many other creatures live in societies and have their own ways of communicating and organising social relationships, we are the only creatures who communicate verbally our thoughts and feelings to each other, gossip together to pass the time of day or tell each other stories and through them relive and share our experiences.

The development of a child's language is closely tied to the maturation of the brain and the abilities the brain supports and enables. At birth your baby's memory span is too short and this ability to organise the sequence of the little sounds that make up words (either to decode meaning or to produce spoken words and sentences) is far too complex for the baby's immature brain to cope with. His brain is, after all, less than half the size of your adult brain – and most of the bits that are missing are those that provide you with the complex infrastructure (memory, fine motor control, random access to information) that enables you to understand the spoken word and to produce it.

This does not mean that children do not start on the complicated business of learning how to speak from an early age: they do. It is the perception of language rather than the production that kicks in first. In an intriguing study carried out in the 1970s, two scientists filmed newborn babies as they listened to various sounds. When, later, they did a frame-by-frame analysis of what the babies did as they listened to people talking, they discovered the babies were moving in synchrony with the rhythms of the speech they were listening to. This squirming dance to the rhythm of voices was unexpected (though perhaps should not have been, because newborn babies have spent months in the womb listening to their mother's voice, and humans find the urge to move to any rhythm almost irresistible). A baby who kicked and stretched in the amniotic fluid to the gentle rhythm of his mother's voice would obviously respond to the pattern of voices he heard after birth. Moving to the rhythm of speech is not the only way a small baby responds to voices. He will turn towards someone speaking in front of him, and soon after birth will also turn to look at anyone speaking off to one side.

When we speak we snatch in a breath and let it out slowly. At other times humans (like most other creatures) blow-breathe: draw air in slowly and push it out fast. Babies change from blow-breathing to snatch-breathing in the early weeks of life. By three months they have switched to the snatch-breathing pattern needed for speech. You will know when it happens because his crying sounds more mature and melodious once he can control the out breath. (And you may begin to interpret different meanings to his cries.) Nor is the preparation of breathing patterns the only way a child prepares for language. From the very beginning he engages in a turn-taking dance with those who care for him: a dance that takes the form of a conversation. You ask him a question – he looks intently back at you maybe moving his lips in answer. You answer with a smile; he smiles back; you ask a question and poke out your tongue; so does he. When parents speak to babies they always leave space for an answer because, if they do not, babies look away and lose interest. Most of the time they answer for the baby, so things go a little like this:

Mother:	*Did you have a nice sleep?*
Baby:	Looks intently while mother pauses
Mother:	*You did?*
Baby:	Looks and squirms
Mother:	*Yes, you did.*

But though he answers back and this has the structure of conversation, a small baby's ability to communicate is limited to a set of facial expressions and bodily postures together with a pattern of noises including crying and gurgling. These tell us the baby's current state – hungry, happy, uncomfortable – but do not inform beyond this. Even when social smiles and other facial expressions are added to the baby's repertoire, babies only match their behaviour to your behaviour – they do not try to share their experiences. We watch, they watch, and we fall in step; but real sharing (of experiences) does not begin until towards the end of the first year. This is when babies start to point at things they want to show us, use gestures to tell us they want to be picked up and begin to look at us to check our reactions to things. Then they use this to guide their own feelings and reactions: to feel afraid *because* we show fear, to be unhappy *because* we are sad. It is at this point that real communication begins. The first questionnaire looks at the precursors to language that tell us when this point is reached.

Matching or Sharing: What Form Does Your Baby's Emotional Relationship Take?

This test is primarily about social referencing but also includes other behaviour – such as the development of mobility – that is closely tied to the beginning of social referencing. Around seven months of age children begin to look to their caregivers for some indication of how they should act and feel, especially how they should act and feel when faced with anything that is unfamiliar to them. Social referencing (as this tendency is called) develops sooner in children who are able to move about on their own. The smiles and gurgles of younger children are a more rudimentary form of communication than social referencing and, although smiles and gurgles set the patterns for turn-taking and basic communication, it is realising that he shares emotions and experiences that drives language development. Why else would he want to speak?

Social referencing helps him to match words to objects. Because we tend to look at (and point to) the things we speak of, children who look where we are looking get a reasonable idea of what the words we use mean. When we look at the cat and say '*Look, a cat*' the emphasis we give to words tells him which words are important. If we pause after saying 'look' and wait until his eyes are on the cat before naming it (as parents naturally do) he hears the word cat while looking at the cat and so gets a good idea of what the word cat means. It is only by exposure to numerous examples of words and objects that children get to know the exact meaning of words. They are helped by a natural tendency to be over-inclusive about meanings: to think, for example, that all little things are babies, or all men are Daddy. They grab a word by its approximate meaning and fine tune its meaning by using it.

Although the roots of language are found in the way the child communicates in his second half year, language explodes properly between his first and third birthday. For most of the second year (between the ages of one and two) he will use one-word utterances (or more often a gesture plus a word), but as his second birthday approaches he begins to use simple, telegraphic two-word sentences. The questionnaire on page 100 looks at the earliest stages in the development of sentences.

1. If you look in the mirror together does your baby

a) Smile and 'talk' to the mirror image?

b) Smile and reach out to pat the mirror image?

2. If you point to something across the room does your baby

a) Look at your fingers?

b) Look where you are pointing?

3. If you are playing with your baby face-to-face and look to one side does he

a) Look at your face? ○

b) Follow your gaze? ○

4. If you shake a rattle to attract your baby's attention does he

a) Look between the rattle and his hand as he reaches for the rattle? ○

b) Look between you and the rattle before or after reaching? ○

5. If you encounter something new does your baby

a) Respond in a fairly consistent way – (depending on his temperament) embracing or rejecting the new? ○

b) Look to you for guidance, then embracing what you embrace, rejecting what you reject? ○

6. If you leave the room does your baby

a) Carry on playing happily? ○

b) Follow you if he can and object if he cannot? ○

7. If you hand your baby to someone he barely knows for a cuddle is he

a) Happy? ○

b) Distraught? ○

8. As your baby plays does he

a) Look up when you call to him? ○

b) Look up at intervals to check on you even if you do not call? ○

9. If your baby is cared for by a new babysitter does he

a) Settle quite happily? ○

b) Protest and cry as you leave? ○

10. If your baby drops a toy from the high chair does he

a) Ignore it and pick up something else to play with? ○

b) Look at the toy, then at you, 'asking' for you to pick it up
for him? ○

11. Is your baby mobile?

a) No. ○

b) Yes. ○

12. Does your baby babble?

a) No. ○

b) Yes. ○

13. Does your baby make a particular noise when he wants attention?

a) No. ○

b) Yes. ○

14. Does your baby lift his arms to be picked up?

a) No. ○

b) Yes. ○

15. Does your baby turn his head away when he does not want food?

a) No. ○

b) Yes. ○

16. Does your baby

a) Make noises when talked to? ○

b) Attempt to imitate the noises you make? ○

17. Does your baby

a) Coo and make throaty noises when he is happy? ○

b) Repeat syllables in strings such as 'Da-da-da' or 'Ma-ma-ma' especially if you encourage him to do so? ○

18. Does your baby respond to his name?

a) No. ○

b) Yes. ○

19. If you play peek-a-boo does your baby

a) Laugh? ○

b) Try to join in? ○

20. If a toy is placed out of reach does your baby

a) Try to reach it?

b) Communicate to you that he wants you to get it for him?

INTERPRETING THE SCORES

❑ **Mainly 'a's. Expected age: children under about six months.** Your child is at the stage where he shares pleasure and emotion with you but communication of emotion is restricted to face-to-face interactions. He has strong emotional feelings and we recognise these by his expressions, but his smiles and frowns, surprised and fearful looks, are a consequence of feeling emotions, not primarily a way of communicating them to us. His expression of emotion and our perception of that emotion is very much in the here and now. He cannot tell us how he felt 10 minutes ago nor how he might feel in 10 minutes' time: something that is quite commonplace for language users. At this stage shared interactions between you and your child occur and persist while you control them. He may engage you and start the game but it will stop if you do not make the effort to maintain it.

❑ **Mixture of 'a's and 'b's. Expected age: children between 6–8 months**. Children are beginning to share emotions and understandings that go beyond themselves and the people, toys and objects that are directly in view. They are beginning to communicate needs – pick me up, do it again – rather than simply expressing the way things are.

❑ **Mainly 'b's. Expected age: children between 8–12 months.** Children are beginning to share experiences and emotions with their caregivers and to look to their caregivers for guidance as to how they should act and feel. Now even after they have reached out for a new toy they will probably check with you that this is okay. Because babies are now beginning to realise that experience is shared they start to communicate their needs and interests to us – asking to be picked up, saying 'No' to another mouthful of food or showing us a cat sitting on the wall.

The Language Test: 10–28 Months

1. Does your child

a) Vocalise to attract attention when he wants something?   ○

b) Say 'More' or, in some recognisable and mutually understood way, ask for more?   ○

c) Ask for exactly what he wants using a short sentence such as 'More milk'?   ○

2. Does your child

a) Wave goodbye when encouraged to do so as someone is about to leave?   ○

b) Say 'Bye-bye' when encouraged? ○

c) Say 'Bye-bye Daddy' or 'Daddy gone' after his Daddy
has left? ○

3. Can your child

a) Point to show you where something is when you ask? ○

b) Indicate he understands your meaning when you say
'Give me' or 'Show me' or 'Where is'? ○

c) Take you to another room to show you where something
is when asked 'Where is your…'? ○

4. Does your child

a) Make one or more animal noises such as 'Moo moo' or
'Woof woof' when he sees a real or toy animal or a picture
of the animal? ○

b) Point to the animals in a book in response to the question
'Where are the…'? ○

c) Name all the animals in his farm book? ○

5. Does your child

a) Vocalise to music? ○

b) Repeat actions that make people laugh? ○

c) Mime actions and repeat the last word of each line of a
familiar action song? ○

6. Can your child

a) Use at least one word meaningfully even if not clearly? ○

b) Use 50 or more words? ○

c) Use 200+ words? ○

7. Does your child

a) Jabber – make noises that imitate the tonal pattern of speech but without any clear or obvious meaning? ○

b) Jabber but with real words embedded in the flow of his jabbering? ○

c) Combine a noun and an adjective ('Big ball') or a noun and a verb ('Gimme juice')? ○

8. Is your child able to

a) Respond to a question with an action such as lifting his arms when asked 'How big are you?'? ○

b) Point to 12 familiar objects on request? ○

c) Carry out actions in response to five action words? ○

9. When sitting on your lap with a book, or wanting a story, does your child

a) Look at picture books – but want to turn pages quickly? ○

b) Hand you a book when he wants a story? ○

c) Listen intently to a simple story about everyday activities? ○

10. Does your child

a) Laugh, chuckle and squeal as he plays? ○

b) 'Talk', 'jabber' or make noises to his toys as he plays? ○

c) Tell toys what to do as he plays such as 'Go sleep' to the teddy he is putting to bed? ○

11. Does your child

a) Respond to you calling his name by asking to be picked up? ○

b) Tell you his name when asked 'Who is my little boy?'? ○

c) Respond with all the names of his family and pets when asked who they are or shown their photographs? ○

12. Does your child

a) Combine at least two syllables in vocal play such as 'Gagoo'? ○

b) Combine two words 'Daddy shoe'? ○

c) Combine three words 'Daddy big shoe'? ○

13. Does your child

a) Point to one body part or move that part when asked, i.e. move or point to his foot when asked 'Where is Andrew's foot?'? ○

b) Point to himself when asked 'Where is Andrew?'? ○

c) Point to a common object when its use is described, 'What do we use to sweep the floor?', 'What do we use to drink tea?'? ⠕

14. Does your child

a) Look towards (or point to) familiar objects when they are named? ⠕

b) Name 12 familiar objects that you point to in his book? ⠕

c) Pick out detail in familiar picture books, 'Where is the mouse hiding?', 'Find me the red flower'? ⠕

15. Does your child

a) Carry out simple directions when these are accompanied by gestures, such as pointing and saying 'Give me a biscuit'? ⠕

b) Imitate the use of simple objects, such as banging with a hammer or using a duster? ⠕

c) Imitate a sequence of activities you show him, such as putting a doll to bed? ⠕

16. Does your child

a) Stop when you say no – at least 75% of the time? ⠕

b) Say no to himself when he is next to something he must not touch or say 'Hot' when next to the radiator? ⠕

c) Sometimes refuse to obey you when you ask him to do
something or have a tantrum when told no? ◌

17. Does your child

a) Look from person to person when people are gossiping
around him? ◌
b) Pull at your jumper when he wants to show you
something? ◌
c) Answer questions and join in a simple conversation with
family and friends? ◌

18. Does your child

a) Shake his head to say no? ◌
b) Say no when asked 'Do you want…'? ◌
c) Say please and thank you if reminded? ◌

19. Does your child

a) Look towards his Daddy when asked 'Where's Daddy?'? ◌
b) Say 'There!' or 'Daddy' when asked 'Where's Daddy?'? ◌
c) Describe in two words where Daddy is when asked,
i.e. 'Daddy gone' or 'Daddy car'? ◌

20. Does your child

a) Copy gestures, such as clapping his hands for pat-a-cake? ◌

b) Spontaneously produce gestures, such as pointing or clapping, i.e. not only in imitation of your gestures? ○

c) Pretend to pour a cup of tea, cook dinner or put a doll to bed? ○

INTERPRETING THE SCORES

❑ **Mainly 'a's. Expected age: children between 10–14 months.** Your child is beginning to understand that he can communicate and that communication is not just restricted to face-to-face interactions. He is beginning to intentionally share his emotions and understanding and to communicate with gestures and sounds. At this stage words are often no more than repeated sounds such as 'Numnum' for food or 'Moo moo' for cow.

❑ **Mixture of 'a's and 'b's. Expected age: children between 12–18 months.** Your child is beginning to use words. He may still use repeated sounds as words, such as 'Woof woof' for dog or 'Brmbrm' for car, but also uses 'real' words. If these are short they often lack endings – he may, for example, say 'Ca' for cat and longer words may simply repeat the first syllable rather than combine two different syllables – such as saying 'Momo' for motorbike. Sometimes he uses two sounds but does not use the word ending – such as 'Bubba' for butter or 'Tratra' for tractor. While most words are a little difficult to follow at this stage, he may have one splendid party piece such as 'Helicopter' or 'Prettyflower'.

❑ **Mainly 'b's. Expected age: children between 16–20 months.** By the time the average child is 18 months he has about 50 words and understands about 500. There are fewer repeated syllables, and because more words have endings they are clearer but he still probably uses 'Moo moo' for cows and leaves the ends off many words. 'Ca' may mean car or cat and although you need to guess from the context which one he means, he is perfectly aware of which one he intended to use.

❑ **Mixture of 'b's and 'c's. Expected age: children between 20–24 months.** By the time he reaches two your child will probably have between 200–300 words and will have started to talk in short telegraphic sentences. His understanding of words far outstrips his ability to produce them – so although he only says 200 words he probably understands 2,000.

❑ **Mainly 'c's. Expected age: children between 24–30 months.** By the time he is 30 months old your child can probably say between 300–600 words and is able to understand between 3,000–6,000 different words. He will be using at least 2–3-word sentences and producing grammatical sentences – although many aspects of grammar are still absent. So he will not, for example, use the little connecting words such as 'an' or 'the' or use different tenses for verbs, or the plural.

How Many Words Does Your Toddler Say?

Surveys suggest that the average English-speaking child uses approximately 10 words or meaningful sounds by the age of 13–14 months; 50 words by the age of 17–18 months and 200–300 words by their second birthday, but there is a huge variation between children. As a general rule of thumb girls are a little more advanced than boys, left-handed children may be a little slower than right-handed children and children in families in which dyslexia is common are often slow to say words and this applies especially to boys. (Their understanding may be normal although production is delayed.) Poor hearing is another reason for slow progress. If you are concerned about your child's progress ask your doctor or health visitor for a developmental and hearing check.

If your child was born prematurely expect progress in terms of *due date* rather than birth date. Note too that for most children the delay is in getting going: once under way, children progress in leaps and bounds. Most children understand about 10 times as many words as they can produce, the most precocious children often have a closer match between understanding and producing words, and the opposite is true for some children whose speech development is delayed.

Counting words is a daunting task. You can get a reasonable daily estimate by listing the words he uses in a five-minute sample, and repeating this half a dozen times throughout the day. Multiply the number of unique words in these six lists by two, then by an estimate of how many hours he spends talking each day. If you multiply this last figure by seven you should get a weekly total, which should approximate to his total word count.

A child with a small vocabulary will tend to repeat many words, while one with a larger vocabulary will not. For this purpose different parts of speech are different words. So 'ship' and 'ships' are two words, so are 'be' and 'been', 'land' and 'landed' and 'go' and 'going'.

TYPICAL WORD COUNT IN CHILDREN OVER 30 MONTHS

3 years	830 words	5 years	2,000 words
3½ years	1,200 words	5½ years	2,200 words
4 years	1,500 words	6 years	2,400 words
4½ years	1,800 words		

 ## Words to Grammar

Once the child has between 100 and 200 words and meaningful sounds, he begins to put words together to form simple sentences. Just as the first words were preceded by meaningful gestures, so the first sentences are preceded by gestures plus words. He might, for example, point to his hat and say 'Alfie', meaning perhaps 'Alfie's hat'.

Sometimes, of course, we get the interpretation wrong. He may mean 'Give me the hat!', and if he does he will probably guide us to the correct interpretation by saying 'No' and 'Hat' or reaching towards the hat and saying 'Hat' in a whining tone until we get the correct message.

Once children begin to replace the gesture with a second word the child makes rapid progression towards fully grammatical sentences. As a rule of thumb most children are putting words together to form two-word sentences by the time they have a vocabulary of 100 words, which for most children is just before their second birthday. There is, however, a huge variation in the speed of language development.

Beginning to use grammar

1. How many different words and meaningful sounds does your child have?

a) 50.

b) Around 300–350.

c) Around 500–600.

2. Does your child put together

a) A word plus a gesture?

b) Two-word sentences?

c) 4–5-word sentences?

3. Does your child ask questions?

a) No. ○

b) By raising intonation at the end of a word. ○

c) Using 'where' and 'what'. ○

4. Does your child express possession ('That's Daddy's car')?

a) By saying 'Daddy' and pointing to the car. ○

b) By saying 'Daddy car'. ○

c) By saying 'That's Daddy's'. ○

5. Does your child express agent-action (Alfie is jumping)?

a) By saying 'Jump'. ○

b) By saying 'Alfie jump'. ○

c) By saying 'Alfie jumping' or 'Alfie is jumping'. ○

6. Does your child express agent-object (read a story)?

a) By bringing you his book and saying 'Book' or 'Story'. ○

b) By bringing a book and saying 'Alfie story' or 'Read story'. ○

c) By bringing a book and saying 'Read me a story'. ○

7. Does your child express action location (come here, play out)?

a) By saying 'Out'. ○

b) By saying 'Play out'. ○

c) By saying 'Can I play out?' ○

8. Does your child express attribution (big book)?

a) By saying 'Big' or 'Big one'. ○

b) By saying 'Big book'. ○

c) By saying 'It's a big book'. ○

9. Does your child express nomination (that chair)?

a) By saying 'Chair'. ○

b) By saying 'That chair'. ○

c) By saying 'In that chair', 'Near that chair', 'It's that chair'. ○

10. Does your child express recurrence (more apple)?

a) By saying 'More'. ○

b) By saying 'More apple'. ○

c) By saying 'More apples'. ○

INTERPRETING THE SCORES

❑ **Mostly 'a's.** Your child is probably under 18 months and like most children of this age is still using holophrases – combining gestures, words and noises to express meaning. Although he is not able to express things clearly he almost certainly understands what he means to say. At this stage in children's development parents usually expand the child's words to make meaning clear. So, for example, when the child gestures towards the apple and says 'More' his parent will reply by saying 'You want more apple?'

or 'Yes, there are more apples in the bowl' – depending on what they think the child means. If the parent does not make the correct interpretation the child is likely to say 'No! More!' Or shake his head and say 'More'. Parents then respond with another interpretation. And so things continue until the parent understands the meaning that the child wishes to convey.

❏ **Mostly 'b's.** Your child is probably approaching his second birthday and is using a combination of gesture and two-word utterances to convey meaning. Most children's utterances combine a limited number of operators (words used rather like verbs) and many more noun-like words. Popular operators are words like 'gimme', 'all-gone', 'that', 'want', 'bye-bye', which the child combines with the names of objects and people.

❏ **Mostly c's.** Your child is probably around two-and-a-half to three and beginning to use a variety of grammatical rules. Between now and his sixth birthday he will master all the subtle rules of the language(s) he speaks.

Elaborating grammar

As children string together more and more words to form longer and more complete sentences they inevitably increase the complexity of the grammatical devices they use. It is these grammatical devices that are absent in one- and two-word utterances. Whether children learn their grammar early or late, it appears in roughly the same order. Tick these off as your child uses them:

1. Expressing temporary duration: 'I walking', 'Jamie jumping', 'Pussy sleeping'. ○

2. Expressing containment: 'In drawer', 'In box'. ○

3. Expressing support: 'On table', 'On bed'. ○

4. Expressing number: 'Two shoes', 'Three chairs'. ○

5. Using the verb 'to be' in full form: 'There it is'. ○

6. Expressing prior occurrence (irregular instances): 'It broke'. ○

7. Expressing possession: 'Mary's hat', 'Adam's shoe'. ○

8. Using articles (a, an, the): 'That a dog', 'That the cat'. ○

9. Expressing prior occurrence (regular examples): 'He walks', 'He does'. ○

10. Using third person (regular use): 'She runs', 'He hops'. ○

11. Using third person (irregular use): 'He does', 'She has'. ○

12. Progressives auxiliary: 'This is going'. ○

13. Using the contracted form of the verb 'to be': 'That's teddy's', 'That's mine'. ○

14. Expressing temporary duration or prior occurrence: 'I'm walking'. ○

15. Using regular past tense: 'I walked'. ○

What does he know about grammar rules?

Just because a child says 'Two teddies' does not mean he has learned to express the plural – that in English we normally do this by adding an 's' to the end of the word. He could simply be copying words he has heard others say. It is only when he applies the rule to words he has never heard before that we know for certain that the rule is understood.

Once a child learns a rule he will – in the initial stages – apply it across the board. So having learned the plural he will apply the rule 'add an s' to lots of irregular instances. He might, for example, refer to 'sheeps', 'feets' or 'foots'. He might also add 'ed' to irregular past tenses like 'ran', 'swam', 'broke' and 'came'. Although he has probably used these words correctly in the past he now says 'runned', 'swimmed', 'breaked' and 'comed'.

When he says 'ran' he may be imitating what he has heard – because this is what you might say – but when he says 'runned' he is not imitating you (you do not use the word), but constructing the past tense by applying the rule of adding 'ed' – even though in this case it is inappropriate.

The easiest way to find out what your child knows about grammar is to listen to him speaking: and when you hear the first examples of a grammatical construction try out the following tests.

KNOWING THE RULE FOR EXPRESSING TEMPORARY DURATION

Take a soft toy or teddy and act out various ways of getting up and about, commenting as you go. So, for example, you might say:

'Here is Teddy going for a walk.'

'Teddy is walking.'

'What is Teddy doing now?'

If he does not say 'walking' tell him the answer. Then put the teddy in a car and say:

'Here is Teddy going for a drive.'

'Teddy is driving.'

'What is Teddy doing now?'

Then take the teddy and do something odd with it – like flying or somersaulting though the air, then say:

'Here is teddy going for a plink.'

Then ask him: 'What is teddy doing?'

Does he say 'plinking'? If he does you know he has learned the rule of adding 'ing' to the end of the word to express temporary duration. It must be the rule because he has never heard anyone say 'plinking'. Plink is a made-up word.

KNOWING THE RULE FOR EXPRESSING THE PLURAL

Take five bits of shaped pasta and say:

'This pasta is called "wump".'

Show him one piece of pasta and say:

'Here is one wump.'

Then take another piece and say:

'Here is another wump'.

Then show him the other three and count:

'One-two-three-four-five.'

Then ask him: 'How many are there?'

If he just says 'five' ask him 'five what?'

If he understands that in English we make the plural by adding 's' he should say 'wumps'.

He must know the rule because he has never heard anyone say 'wumps' because wump is a made-up word.

KNOWING THE RULE FOR EXPRESSING THE REGULAR PAST TENSE

Take a soft toy or teddy and walk him across the table saying:

'Teddy is walking.'

Then ask: 'Did Teddy run or did he walk? What did he do?'

He should answer that Teddy 'walked'. Now move the teddy in a different way and say:

'Teddy is blogging.'

Then ask: 'Did Teddy blog or did he plunk?'

Does he say 'Teddy plunked'? In other words, did he add the 'ed' to 'plunk'? If he does this you know he understands that to make a past tense you need to add an 'ed'. He must know the rule because he has never heard anyone else say 'plunked'; it is a made-up word.

Top Tips

1. Talk to him frequently. This is important as, even when he is too young to understand what you say, he can learn the rules of turn taking.

2. Give him time to answer – even when he is too young to formulate the answer – but more importantly when he is able to answer you.

3. Listen to him: do not jump in too quickly.

4. Get down to his level. Whenever it is possible to do so, face him when you talk.

5. Eat together at the table. This encourages face-to-face conversation.

6. Expand and clarify what he says.

7. Practice tailoring your speech to your child's understanding, using a higher pitch and short, simple sentences.

8. Find time for a chat.

9. Read books. It is important training in story telling.

10. Use rhyme and rhythm – reading rhyming books like *The Cat in the Hat* helps him hear the little sounds that make up words. This is important for speaking and later for learning to read.

Chapter 4

Testing Knowledge of Self and Others

Understanding Who She Is

At birth a young baby does not understand where she stops and where the rest of the world begins. Why should she? The womb is a dimly lit and watery world that changes little: deep red when her mother's skin is exposed to light, otherwise dark; all she feels is the fluid around her, her own body and the edges of the sac that contains her. She hears the constant sound of her mother's heart and the gush of her blood. Up to the moment she enters the world it is as if she is an extension of her mother's body; food and oxygen arrive in her bloodstream and waste products are taken away by the same route. The only changes she perceives are her mother's movements and the sound of her voice and, since she has no control over these, there is no reason for her to think they are separate from her or under her control.

All this changes at birth. Now what she sees depends upon where she looks, and nutrition and excretion depend on the action of her own body. Over the first few months she learns that her hands and feet belong to her, that her cries attract her mother's attention and her smiles her mother's voice. She begins to realise she has the ways and means to make things happen.

Knowing she is separate from you

1. Does your child watch

a) If someone moves directly into her line of sight? ○

b) AND turn to follow their movement with her eyes? ○

2. If you say 'Hey, baby' does your child

a) Look at you? ○

b) Widen her eyes, tilt her head up and smile broadly? ○

3. Has your baby laughed yet?

a) No. ○

b) Yes. ○

4. Does your baby

a) Glance at her hands if they come into view? ○

b) Watch her hands intently if they come into view? ○

5. Does your baby

a) Become excited if her arms happen to knock a toy and make it move? ○

b) Try to repeat an action that makes something move? ○

6. Does your baby

a) Smile in her sleep? ○
b) Lock eyes with you and smile when she sees your face? ○

7. Can you tell what your baby's cries mean? Does she 'cry on purpose' to make things happen or to let you know her needs?

a) No. ○
b) Yes. ○

8. Is your baby able to find the nipple?

a) Only if you touch her cheek so that she opens her
    mouth and turns towards you. ○
b) By rooting for the breast without your help. ○

9. If you place a finger in each hand does your baby

a) Automatically grasp them so firmly that you could lift her? ○
b) Grasp but not firmly enough to be lifted very far? ○

10. When resting does your baby

a) Prefer a foetal position? ○
b) Spread out her arms and legs? ○

11. Does your baby suck?

a) While feeding.

b) While feeding AND between feeds she also sucks her
thumb or her dummy?

12. Does your baby repeat actions that bring pleasure such as thumb-sucking, exchanging facial expressions or looking for (and finding) her mobile?

a) No.

b) Yes.

INTERPRETING THE SCORES

❑ **Mostly 'a's.** Your baby is probably under two months old. She does not yet realise that she is separate from the world around her or that she can have any influence on the world.

❑ **Mixture of 'a's and 'b's.** Your child is probably around 6–9 weeks old and is beginning to realise where her body stops and the rest of the world begins and that she can influence the world about her, including the people in her life.

❑ **Mostly 'b's.** Your baby is probably around 8–12 weeks old and has learned that she has some control over her body – she can purposely look in order to see certain things and make her hands move and reach out to explore, which means she now knows where her body stops and the rest of the world begins.

What Makes Your Baby Smile?

Here are some simple experiments to examine what makes a baby smile. When looking at stage one smiles, bear in mind that the first smiles occur at a more or less fixed date from conception: so babies who are early for dates smile later and those who were born late for dates smile sooner than average. Average is around six weeks of age.

FIRST SMILES: APPROXIMATELY 4–10 WEEKS

In the initial stages babies smile in their sleep. These early smiles do not light up their faces (they may not even light up all of their lips: sometimes these first smiles are confined to one side of the face). The very first smiles occur when babies move from one state of arousal to another, but later smiles also occur when sleeping babies hear high-pitched sounds.

❏ Try raising your voice or ringing a tinkling bell close to your sleeping baby.

FIRST VOLUNTARY SMILES: APPROXIMATELY 6–13 WEEKS

Some time between about six and 13 weeks babies give their first waking smiles – smiles that are beginning to really light up their faces. Now high-pitched voices work when babies are awake and so do nodding heads.

❏ Try looking your baby in the eye, shaking your head and saying in a high-pitched voice, 'Hello, my little darling.'

❏ You could also try ringing a bell or shaking a rattle where she can see it – especially a rattle with a face drawn on it.

FIRST SOCIAL SMILES: APPROXIMATELY 10–20 WEEKS

At around three months nodding heads lose their charm and, although babies still like a higher-pitched voice, what now brings on the biggest smiles is a stationary face (especially, but not only, a familiar one) that is smiling back at them. Now her smiles light up her entire face, eyes engage, mouth opens and eyebrows rise.

❏ Check out the nodding moving head and the rattle with a face, then

❏ Try looking your baby in the eye and talking to her.

LAUGHTER: APPROXIMATELY 16–28 WEEKS

Laughter follows from these really broad, full-faced social smiles. At first babies laugh in response to sounds and touches; later laughter is elicited by surprising and complex situations such as playing peek-a-boo or jiggling her on your knee and letting her drop suddenly between your legs. By laughing at the unexpected your child tells you that she knows (she has learned and she remembers) what to expect. Before the 28 weeks is up she may well be letting you know that when you play 'This is the way the ladies ride', she knows the old man is about to go 'down into the ditch', and when you play 'This little piggy', her foot will be held out ready for you to start.

- ☐ Try showing your baby toys that disappear and reappear.
- ☐ Try kissing her tummy.
- ☐ Try playing peek-a-boo.
- ☐ Try swooping in with a toy duck to peck at her tummy.
- ☐ Try tickling her toes or playing 'This little piggy'.
- ☐ Try playing 'This is the way the ladies ride' or 'Leg over, leg over, the dog went to Dover'.
- ☐ Laughter is infectious – and your baby is easily infected! Just laugh and she will join in.

Social Referencing: the Second Six Months

Even when social smiles and laughter are added to the baby's repertoire, babies do not fully share their experiences with us. We share because *we* fall in step with *their* needs and interests. We lure them into laughter, we comfort their fears, we interpret their needs and start the conversations. The real and obvious sharing of experience happens towards the end of the first year when babies begin to use body language to communicate need, and point to things they wish to share with us. We can see the subtle beginnings of these skills from about seven months (even earlier in babies who crawl early). At about this time babies start to use gestures to tell us what they want

– such as raising their arms to tell us they want to be picked up or putting out a foot when they want us to play 'This little piggy' again.

At the same time something quite subtle happens: babies begin to look at us to check our reactions to events before they act. In other words they use our response to a situation as a guide to their own feelings and reactions: to feel afraid *because* we show fear, or feel happy and secure *because* we are laughing and smiling. Babies mirror our facial responses – they follow smiles with smiles, eyebrow raises with eyebrow raises – which is perhaps what is happening in emotional terms. Psychologists have shown that if you hold a certain facial expression (even if someone pushes and pulls your face into that expression) you begin to feel the emotion your face depicts. All those old sayings about smiling and putting on a brave face have more than a crumb of truth about them.

Has your baby started social referencing?

Below is a questionnaire that examines social referencing (the name given to this checking of others' feelings). The test measures how readily children share emotions and experiences. Once your baby begins to understand that you have a separate identity from her (which happens at about seven months of age), she will begin to look to you for some indication of how she should act and feel. Especially how she should act and feel when faced with anything that is unfamiliar to her. Social referencing develops sooner in mobile children.

1. If you point to something across the room does your baby

a) Look at your fingers? ◯

b) Look where you are pointing? ◯

2. If your child drops a toy does she look for it?

a) No. ◯

b) Yes. ◯

3. Does your child like to play peek-a-boo?

a) No. ◯

b) Yes. ◯

4. When playing games in which your child rides on your knee ('This is the way the ladies ride'; 'Leg over, leg over') does she in any way indicate that she wants more?

a) No. ◯

b) Yes. ◯

5. When your child is riding on your knee playing games which include a fall between your legs ('This is the way the ladies ride'), does she look at you in anticipation before she falls 'down into the ditch'?

a) No. ○

b) Yes. ○

6. If you are playing with your baby face-to-face, then look to one side, does she

a) Look at your face? ○

b) Follow your gaze? ○

7. If you shake a rattle to attract your baby's attention does she

a) Look between the rattle and her hand as she reaches for the rattle? ○

b) Look between you and the rattle before or after reaching? ○

8. If you encounter something new does your baby

a) Respond in a fairly consistent way – dependent on her temperament, either embracing or rejecting the new? ○

b) Look to you for guidance, then embracing what you embrace, rejecting what you reject? ○

9. As your child plays does she

a) Look up when you call to her? ○

b) Look up at intervals to check on you even if you do not call? ○

10. If a toy is placed out of reach does your child

a) Try to reach it? ○

b) Communicate to you that she wants you to get it for her? ○

11. Does your baby recognise

a) Her main caregiver? ○

b) All the members of her family? ○

12. Is your child

a) Happy to be with strangers? ○

b) Beginning to be shy and anxious with strangers? ○

13. Does your baby

a) Kick and show pleasure when you talk to her? ○

b) React to the tone of your voice: happy when you are
happy, uneasy if you are angry or upset? ○

14. When giving your child food does she

a) Open her mouth as the spoon approaches? ○

b) Sometimes refuse to open her mouth? ○

15. Does your child understand NO!

a) No. ○

b) Yes. ○

INTERPRETING THE SCORES

❑ **Mainly 'a's. Expected age: children under 5–7 months.** Your child is at the stage where she shares pleasure and emotion with you but the communication of emotion is restricted to face-to-face interactions. She has strong emotional feelings that you recognise but her expression of emotion and your perception of that emotion is very much in the here and now. She cannot tell you how she felt 10 minutes ago nor how she might feel in 10 minutes' time.

❑ **Mixture of 'a's and 'b's. Expected age: children between 6–8 months.** Children are now beginning to share emotions and understandings that go beyond themselves and the people, toys and objects that are directly in view. They are starting to interactively tell you what they want and how they feel.

❑ **Mainly 'b's. Children between 8–12 months.** Children are beginning to share experiences and emotions with their caregivers and to look to their caregivers for guidance as to how they should act and feel. Communication has moved right into the forefront. They want to show you – and in time will become angry and frustrated when you do not understand (which is what the 'terrible twos' are all about!)

Fear of Strangers and Separation Anxiety

In their second half-year of life children become fearful of strangers – and this includes people like grandparents they have not seen for some time. Fear of strangers can develop as early as four months but usually does not happen before six months. Here are the norms for the age at which the behaviour is first shown.

Age of baby	Percentage who first show fear of strangers
21–24 weeks	0%
25–28 weeks	16%
29–32 weeks	25%
33–36 weeks	32%
37–40 weeks	11%
41–44 weeks	6%
45–48 weeks	3%
49–78 weeks	5%

WHAT DOES THIS TELL US ABOUT OUR BABY?

You cannot be afraid of strangers until you know who the strangers are: so we know that when babies begin to show this fear (and when later they become fearful and clinging in strange places) they remember their own family. They know you and remember you not just when they see you, but also when they are looking at someone else. It may seem a simple thing, but if you have a tiny little memory (as babies do) it is not. To be afraid of this stranger she needs to look beyond the stranger's smiling face and their cooing voice and realise that this is not one of the faces she knows and loves. This means in turn that she is beginning to understand that there is only one you (we saw how to test this in Chapter 2, page 81) and that you do not just disappear when you move out of sight.

Separation anxiety – the fear expressed by the child when left alone by the parent or caregiver – happens a little later when children have fully understood that carers and loved ones continue to exist when she cannot see them. Children suffering from separation anxiety cry, cling and try to regain contact when carers leave them. Separation anxiety begins somewhat later than fear of strangers – starting at around 36 weeks, reaching a peak at around 78 weeks (18 months), and declines thereafter. It tends to be more variable – especially in children who are cared for by a number of different people. Initially, children are anxious and cling even when their mothers leave them in familiar places. Gradually the clinginess becomes notable mainly when the child is somewhere new – which tells us she can now compare home and away from home.

Observing the Development of Empathy and Social Understanding

This is an observational test for children between 10 months and 30 months that uses various indicators to assess whether babies understand how others think and feel.

1. Does your child cry if she hears others cry?

a) Yes. ○

b) No. ○

2. Does your child try to comfort others when they are distressed – even if the action (like offering you her dummy) is not always appropriate?

a) No. ○

b) Yes. ○

3. Does your child express her concern (even with only a stroke or a sloppy kiss) if you are ill or upset?

a) No. ○

b) Yes. ○

4. When your child holds out a toy to another child does she pay any attention to whether the other child can see it?

a) No. ○

b) Yes. ⚪

5. When playing with a younger child does your child adjust her behaviour to take the age difference into account?

a) No. ⚪
b) Yes. ⚪

6. Does your child share her toys without too many upsets?

a) Yes. ⚪
b) No. ⚪

7. Does your child spontaneously help with chores?

a) No. ⚪
b) Yes. ⚪

8. Does your child sometimes take a toy she wants even when another child is playing with it?

a) Yes. ⚪
b) No. ⚪

9. Does your child offer toys to other children?

a) No. ⚪
b) Yes. ⚪

10. If your child is in conflict with other children does she

a) Grab what she wants? ◌

b) Try to negotiate or cajole the other child into letting her have what she wants? ◌

11. Does your child sometimes hit other children – but without obvious malice?

a) Yes. ◌

b) No. ◌

12. Does your child sometimes push or bite other children?

a) Yes. ◌

b) No. ◌

13. Does your child sometimes grab your earrings even though you have told her it hurts?

a) Yes. ◌

b) No. ◌

14. Does your child pull other people's hair?

a) Yes. ◌

b) No. ◌

15. Does your child offer you a lick of her ice-cream (or a piece of her banana if that is her treat)?

a) No.   ○

b) Yes.   ○

INTERPRETING THE SCORES

❑ **Mostly 'a's.** At 10 months children like to be with other children but are trapped within their own thoughts and feelings. They have no real understanding that other children are separate people, so they do not understand they must check whether the other child is looking before they offer toys, or that another child might be upset if they take away their plaything. The up-side of this is that they are not very upset when someone takes a toy from them, the downside is that they do not understand they should not hit or bite. (If it does not hurt them to hit or bite, it will not hurt anyone else!)

❑ **Mostly 'b's.** By the time children reach 30 months they are beginning to understand they must take other people's behaviour into consideration – even though they are not yet skilled at doing so. They check that other children can see toys they offer to them and are more inclined to negotiate before taking a toy from another child. They may not understand that our thoughts and feelings are separate from theirs (that comes later) but they do know that certain actions make us unhappy and make others cry.

Becoming Interested in Other People

The family is the centre of a baby's world, and although this does not change as babies become toddlers, they inevitably begin to show interest in people outside the home and family – particularly people their own size. Children's interest in other children waxes and wanes in the early years: as babies they love to see other babies; as they approach their first birthday they like to touch, babble-talk and grin at other babies; but soon after their first birthday their interest wanes and they switch from people to things. At 13 months they may be more interested in the toys at mother and baby group than the children playing with them. It is a short phase. By 15 months most toddlers are back on the social trail, able and willing to imitate the actions of other children. They love games, like hide and seek and follow my leader, and songs with actions; these help them form connections between themselves, adults and other children.

Testing whether she understands other people's emotions

The classic test that shows that children understand how others feel uses pictures of children in a number of situations (at a birthday party, with a dog running away, where someone is spoiling a game, when the child gets lost, when her mother's hair turns green) and then asks the child how the person in the picture feels and why they feel that way.

What you need

❑ A picture book telling a happy story or a photo of children at a birthday party.

❑ A picture book telling a sad story or a photo or drawing of a dog running away.

❑ A story about a little child getting lost, or a drawing or photo of a child alone.

What to do

Tell the child the story or show her the picture and tell the story:

❑ Show her the picture of the party, saying, 'This is Sally's birthday party. Look at the presents her friends have brought her.' (Or 'Look at her lovely birthday tea' if that is what is in the picture.) Then ask, 'How does Sally feel when her friends arrive with presents?'

❑ Show her the dog running away and say, 'This is Joey. He is Sally's dog. He is running away. He will get lost and never come back.' Then ask, 'How will Sally feel when she hears her dog has run away?'

❑ Show her the picture of the child by herself and say, 'This is Sally. She has lost her Mummy and is all by herself.' Then ask, 'How does Sally feel when she finds herself all alone and cannot find her Mummy?'

What you should expect to find

At the age of two, most children will say that Sally is happy at her birthday party, but they are unlikely to be able to understand unhappy emotions such as fear or sadness. By the time they are 4–5 years old they can understand how children feel in more negative situations. This is a test you might like to repeat as your child grows up.

Terrible Twos

The terrible twos are the downside of a very special time: a time when good and bad emotions are at the forefront of your child's behaviour. Children do not have tantrums because they are frustrated: they have them because they are frustrated with you. The onset of tantrums and stubborn behaviour tells us that a child has reached the stage where she fully understands the power of communication – and just wishes you were always completely cooperative!

The first test asks you to examine your child's last tantrum – the second test asks you to say how most tantrums occur.

Looking at tantrums

1. Was your child's last tantrum predictable?

a) No, it came out of the blue.

b) Yes and no – I could see she was getting upset.

c) Yes – she had been in a bad mood for a time. She was just trying to goad me. She was asking for the impossible. ○

2. How long did it last?

a) A minute or two – no more. ○
b) A few minutes. ○
c) Five minutes or more. ○

3. How did it start?

a) Suddenly. She was off – screaming, stamping, falling over, etc. ○
b) She wound up to it and then suddenly lost control. ○
c) She was in a difficult mood, she shouted 'No', screamed, stamped and then lost control. ○

4. How did it end?

a) As if nothing had happened. ○
b) She was a bit sad and sorry but only for a moment. ○
c) She remained sad and sorry and needed comforting. ○

5. When was the previous tantrum?

a) The same day. ○
b) The day before. ○
c) The same week. ○

INTERPRETING THE SCORES

❏ **Mostly 'a's.** Your child is probably under two-and-a-half. At this age tantrums arrive out of the blue, flare up and die down. Then it is as if nothing has happened. Probably because at this age children still live very much in the moment.

❏ **Mostly 'b's.** Your child is probably between two-and-a-half and three-and-a-half. Tantrums are now less isolated from her other behaviour; they are more predictable and she is beginning to feel the aftermath – to be sad and sorry and in need of comfort.

❏ **Mostly 'c's.** Your child is probably over three-and-a-half. Tantrums are much more predictable – more often an exaggeration of a negative mood, which is likely to continue after the tantrum is over. She will need forgiveness and comfort.

Tantrums are about relationships

1. Who is with (in charge of) your child when she has tantrums?

a) Mother. ⭕

b) Parents, close family and regular carers. ⭕

c) Strangers, teachers, play-leaders or those she knows less well. ⭕

2. Who is with (in charge of) your child when she has the most severe tantrums?

a) Mother. ⭕

b) Parents, close family and regular carers. ○

c) Strangers, teachers, play-leaders or those she knows less well. ○

3. If you construct a time-with-child by tantrum rate (a tantrum/person/hour rate) who tops the list? Who does she have most tantrums with?

a) Mother. ○

b) Parents, close family and regular carers. ○

c) Strangers, teachers, play-leaders or those she knows less well. ○

4. Where does your child have most of her tantrums?

a) At home or in the car. ○

b) At the shops, at friends' houses or in places where whoever is caring for her is busy. ○

c) Everywhere – she does not have a 'favourite place'. ○

5. Does what your child is doing make tantrums more likely?

a) They are more likely if she is being confined in a place where she cannot see us – a car seat, a pushchair, etc. ○

b) They are more common when she is frustrated by things that go wrong – such as getting her pants on backwards or her socks with the heel upwards. ○

c) No. ○

6. Does your child have more tantrums at certain times of day?

a) Yes – especially mornings and early evenings when I am busy.

b) Yes, at times when she is tired.

c) No.

7. Does your mood affect your child?

a) Sometimes – especially if I am busy or distracted.

b) Occasionally – if I am particularly unhappy or distracted.

c) Never.

8. Does what you are doing make tantrums more likely?

a) Yes – they are more likely when I am busy, talking to other people or distracted.

b) Sometimes – if I am busy, with other people or distracted.

c) No.

9. Does your child ever have tantrums when you are about to leave her – at day care or nursery, or if you are going out and leaving her with a baby-sitter?

a) Yes, often.

b) Sometimes.

c) Never.

10. Can you distract your child before the tantrum starts?

a) Yes. ○

b) Sometimes – but most tantrums come out of the blue. ○

c) No. ○

INTERPRETING THE SCORES

❑ **Mostly 'a's.** Tantrums are about relationships – as your answers show. Almost all children have tantrums with those they love the best and in places they love most and where they feel most secure. Your child has a very close attachment with you.

❑ **Mostly 'b's.** As for 'Mostly 'a's', your child has formed a number of close attachments with family and friends.

❑ **Mostly 'c's.** Very few children fall into this class. If your child is over two and ALSO shows little evidence of social referencing AND is very late speaking, you should mention this to your doctor or health visitor. It could (but does not necessarily) indicate that there may be problems.

 # Understanding and Defining Who She Is

Self-definition grows from the child's ability to understand the world and from emotional understanding of those she loves, and theirs of her. It is perhaps easiest to understand as a construction based on observable aspects of the child. Try asking your child to tell you all about herself. At the age of three, with a little prompting, she might say something like:

'My name is Molly, I am a girl.'

'I live in my house in Windsor Road.'

'My baby is Jamie, my cat is Pumpkin.'

'I have a blue coat and a red bike.'

'My best friend is Nishma and my second best friend is Amy.'

This way of defining oneself is sometimes called the categorical or single representation self. This means that the child thinks of herself in terms of isolated facts ('My cat is Pumpkin', 'I have a blue coat') and, when asked to describe herself, her description jumps about from fact to fact without any logical order or sense of what may be more important. Her thinking (like most preschoolers' thinking) tends to be all-or-none, black-or white. So she loves or hates, rather than feeling indifferent or unconcerned as adults do; and just as she understands positive emotions better than negative ones, she describes the positive aspects of her abilities. She will tell you she is good at jumping and swimming but will fail to tell you she cannot catch a ball. (As we grow up we are more inclined to focus on the negative as you might well see if you described yourself.) She cannot imagine having two emotions at the same time – such as feeling happy and a bit scared.

By the time your child is five her description of herself will link one aspect of her behaviour with other related aspects: 'I am good at drawing and colouring', 'I am good at kicking and scoring goals', but she will still categorise herself by the positive aspects of her character and see these in black and white terms.

Testing her understanding of self and others: the early preschool child

1. When with other children does your child

a) Play in parallel – sitting close, but with each child doing their 'own thing'? ○

b) Share simple domestic play – such as cooking in the kitchen corner? ○

c) Engage in pretence games in which each child has a character to play? ○

2. When you arrive at childcare/nursery/at a friend's house does your child

a) Fuss for a moment but accept that you will leave or be otherwise engaged? ○

b) Greet people if reminded? ○

c) Greet everyone? ○

3. If you talk about your child day does she

a) Rely on you to remember what happened and add comments to indicate she understands and remembers?

b) Correct you if you get a detail wrong?

c) Tell you what she has been doing?

4. If playing with a teddy or a doll does your child

a) Hug or carry it about?

b) Put the teddy or doll to bed?

c) Engage in prolonged domestic play – dressing the doll, combing her hair, etc?

5. When playing pretend games does your child

a) Copy simple actions such as pretending to use an electric iron or feed a teddy?

b) Play through a simple scene such as cooking in her kitchen?

c) Act out characters and elaborate stories when alone – and act out roles in games with other children?

6. If shown family photographs does your child

a) Fail to recognise family members?

b) Recognise family members and familiar adults?

c) Recognise herself?

7. If asked can your child

a) Tell you whether the child in a picture you show her is a boy or a girl? ○

b) Tell you whether she is a boy or a girl? ○

c) Understand that gender does not change – that the gender she is now will be the same when she grows up (that girls do not ever grow up to be daddies and that if she is a girl now, she was not a boy baby)? ○

8. If given a choice of toys/activities does your child

a) Select just any she enjoys playing with? ○

b) Select the most sex-appropriate toys? ○

c) Select the toys/activities her friends are playing? ○

9. When you arrive at a friend's house does your child

a) Cling? ○

b) Remain in the same room and check you are watching out for her? ○

c) Go off and play with the other children? ○

10. Does your child

a) Copy what you do? ○

b) Imitate/pretend to be you? ○

c) Pretend/imitate what the same sex parent does? ○

11. Does your child act as if police helmets and Batman outfits are

a) Dressing-up clothes? ○

b) Boys' dressing-up clothes? ○

c) Dressing-up clothes that girls should not play with even
   in private? ○

12. Who does your child play with?

a) Family and older children and those who invite her into
   the game. ○

b) As above but she also has a current friend or friends – but
   these change week by week. ○

c) She has one or two good friends and prefers to play with
   them. ○

13. Will your child

a) Talk to parents and other close family members? ○

b) Talk with family and with other children? ○

c) Contribute to adult conversations? ○

14. When getting dressed does your child

a) Wear what she is given? ○

b) Have favourite clothes? ○

c) Choose to wear what other children wear? ○

15. When you are reunited after parting does your child

a) Only tell you what she has been doing if you ask – and
   then without detail?   ○

b) Tell you what she has been doing – but do so as if you
   shared her experience?   ○

c) Explain as if she understands you did not share the
   experience?   ○

INTERPRETING THE SCORES

❑ **Mostly 'a's.** Your child is probably about two. She is at the early
  stages of socialisation, a time when her skills are mainly confined
  to family, caregivers and your close friends. She does not yet know
  how to make friends although she can join the games of older
  children. She cannot yet put herself into anyone else's shoes and
  her understanding of herself (and of you) is stuck in the here and
  now. She might, for example, think she will marry Daddy when
  she grows up. She knows she will grow up (as a fact without any
  real understanding) but does not realise you will change too.

❑ **Mostly 'b's.** Your child is probably between three and four. She
  is beginning to make friends and play with other children. She
  is still unable to put herself in other children's shoes but has learned
  to share (sometimes) and not to hit other children (most of the
  time) because that gets her into trouble. She knows she is a girl
  – but may still think she can be a daddy when she grows up. She

likes to play with other girls and chooses sex-appropriate toys, games and activities.

❏ **Mostly 'c's.** Your child is at least four-and-a-half (probably a little older) and is now able to put herself into other people's shoes. She understands you do not share her experiences unless you are with her. She knows she always was, is and will be female but may none the less feel that if she puts a Superman outfit on she might turn into a boy. She is beginning to understand society's rules – and to keep to them even when no one is watching her.

Does your child have a theory of mind?

Small children do not understand that we do not see what they see, experience what they experience or feel what they feel. This sort of knowledge is called a theory of mind, or TOM for short. TOM is the understanding that we each have our own private thoughts, that we know only what we see and hear or what others tell us. TOM is the basis of empathy (putting ourselves in others' shoes) and sympathy (trying to understand how others must feel) as well as deception. Obviously we cannot deceive someone if we think they see and hear exactly what we do. TOM does not develop until relatively late in the preschool years.

It is this lack of TOM that makes your child so transparent: it is hard to deceive until you understand that you can; hard to do so successfully until you can think 'If I do/say that, he will think that

I…'. If she comes home from nursery school saying, 'You know that girl I was playing with…?' even though you were at work and some-one else took her to nursery, you know she does not yet have a TOM. When she comes home saying, 'You know that girl who goes to my school and lives near the shop – the one whose Mummy works in the fish shop? Well, I was playing with her today', you know she now has a TOM. Another sign that TOM is developing is that she starts to use strategies when playing games – or tricks her younger siblings into leaving her with the thing she wants most.

Most four-year-olds will fail 'theory of mind' tests, and many five-year-olds will also fail. Autistic children will not pass these tests until they are very much older and may have difficulty with them even when they are adults. The two tests below are the classic ways of testing whether a child has a theory of mind. They both rely on the child being able to understand that only those who see some-thing happen will know that some deception has occurred.

THE SMARTIE TEST

This test will show whether your child understands that other people do not share her thoughts and feelings.

You will need

❑ An empty box or container that clearly depicts what should be inside. The test is called 'the Smartie test' because it originally used the tubes for sugar-coated chocolate sweets. If you cannot get a Smartie tube choose something the child is familiar with – a packet for raisins, an ice-cream tub or a yoghurt pot with a lid would do. The two important points are that she should not be able to see into the box and she must know what is normally in the box.

❑ You will also need something surprising to put in the box. Pencils were used in the original test but you could choose spoons, crayons, even pasta: anything, providing the child is able to recognise and name these when you show them to her – but don't do this yet! She must not see what is in the box until you are ready.

❑ You will also need a teddy or doll who will be deceived.

What to do

❑ First put the pencils in the Smartie box. Don't let her see you do this. Put the lid back so she cannot see what is in the box.

❑ Sit close to the child and put the teddy next to her. Now hold out the Smartie box. Ask her what is in the box. Then show the box to Teddy and ask what Teddy thinks is in the box. She should answer 'Smarties' both times.

❑ Now say Teddy is going to hide outside the door, and remove him from the room.

❑ After Teddy has gone, tip whatever is in the box out so she can see and ask her what was really in the box. She should answer 'Pencils'. Now return the pencils to the box and replace the lid.

❑ Bring Teddy back into the room and ask your child, 'What does Teddy think is in the box?'

Children without a TOM: if your child does not yet understand that Teddy can only know things he has directly experienced – and thus cannot know about the pencils because he was out of the room when you showed them to the child, she will say 'Pencils'.

Children with a TOM: if your child understands that Teddy can only know what he has directly experienced and thus cannot know about the pencils since he was out of the room when the box was opened she will say 'Smarties'.

THE SALLY ANNE TEST

This test will also show whether your child understands that other people do not share her thoughts and feelings.

You will need

❑ Two dolls or stuffed toys each with a name. The original test used two dolls: one called Sally, the other Anne.

❑ A bag or basket for one doll to carry that contains a precious item – such as a ring or a bar of chocolate. In the original test the precious item was placed in a basket and covered with a cloth.

❑ You also need somewhere obvious (such as under a cushion) to hide the precious object.

What you do

❑ Sit close to the child and sit the two dolls next to you. Give Sally the basket. Ask your child what each doll thinks is in Sally's basket. Both dolls should know about the precious object. If necessary, show the object to the dolls and say, 'Look, Sally has a ring in her basket'.

❑ Now say Sally has to go outside the door. She must leave the basket behind.

❑ Now Anne plays a trick. She takes the precious object from the basket and hides it under the cushion.

❑ Now Sally comes back.

❑ Ask your child, 'Where does Sally think her precious object is?'

Children without a TOM: if your child does not understand that Sally can only know things she has directly experienced – and thus cannot know that Anne has hidden her precious object while she was out of the room, she will say 'Under the cushion'.

Children with a TOM: if your child understands that Sally only knows about things she directly experiences – and thus cannot know that Anne hid her precious object while she was out of the room, she will say 'In the basket'.

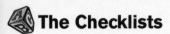

The Checklists

The checklists below follow the child's development over the first five years. They are based on a number of checklists compiled by developmental psychologists who recorded what young children could do at particular ages. They show what the average child can do by a certain age. The lists are arranged in roughly the order that behaviours unfold in the average child. It is unlikely that your child will do things in exactly the order shown. You will find below, in roughly the order they occur, checklists for self-help and care taking: eating, toilet training and dressing.

Checklist for social behaviour

Babies are totally egocentric; they demand attention and expect to get it now – as befits such a helpless bundle. They are incapable of doing things for themselves: they HAVE to make demands if they are to survive. They have a two-pronged attack – they engage our love with smiles and adoring looks, and they let us know by their tears and unhappiness that they need our help. In the first years children must learn to fit into the pattern of their families and into the wider society: to do what that society – and particularly their immediate family – expects of them. A child's capacity for social understanding develops over time, which means, as with motor development, we can construct a checklist for social behaviours.

The list below shows roughly the order in which various aspects of social behaviour develop. There is a little more variability in this list because social behaviours are more dependent on social learning and are more likely to be influenced by the child's temperament.

On average girls develop social skills sooner than boys – but this is not written in stone. There is more variation amongst girls than there is between girls and boys. A child's social development is dependent on her temperament (see Chapter 5) and on the social situation in which she is brought up. Practice makes perfect and imitation plays an important role. So children who grow up in outgoing families often become more skilled. Those who have older siblings find it easier to get on with other children (they have after all been doing this from the cradle), while only children often find it easier to get on with adults.

This test examines the child's social understanding. The other side of social development is the gradual understanding of social norms, conventions and skills, all of which make the child independent.

To carry out this test simply tick everything your child can do. Since the list is constructed in approximately the order in which behaviours develop, it can also tell you what she is likely to do next. When you run out of ticks have a look at the key on page 162.

1. Does she watch you if you move into her bubble of vision?   ◌

2. Does she smile – little windy smiles?   ◌

3. Does she 'answer back' when you talk to her? ◯

4. If you poke your tongue out does she copy you? ◯

5. Is she happy to be passed from person to person? ◯

6. Is she calmed by you picking her up? ◯

7. Does she recognise you? ◯

8. Does she watch her hands? ◯

9. Does she reach out to touch you? ◯

10. Does she cry when left alone? ◯

11. Does she wave her arms and legs, and coo when she sees you? ◯

12. If sitting in front of the mirror does she reach for the baby she sees? ◯

13. When doing things together does she seek eye contact? ◯

14. Is she becoming shy in the company of strangers? ◯

15. Can she tell if you are cross? ◯

16. Can she play peek-a-boo? ◯

17. Does she offer things to you (but may not release them)? ◯

18. Does she lift her arms to be picked up? ◯

19. Will she raise her arms if you ask how big she is? ◯

20. Does she hug and kiss those she loves? ◯

21. Does she know her name? ◯

22. Does she refuse to go to strangers? ◯

23. Does she look up from what she is doing to find you? ◯

24. Does she look where you look? ◯

25. Does she 'join in', making noises, laughing, when you play together? For example, is she ready to ride before you start to jog her on your knee? ○

26. Does she cling when you leave her? ○

27. Is she beginning to communicate using noises and gestures? ○

28. Does she wave bye-bye? ○

29. Does she have a comforter – a teddy or a blanket or dummy that calms and brings security when she is sad and is with her when she sleeps? ○

30. In a strange place does she move away to play but look up for reassurance or come back to you often? ○

31. If you do something (such as banging the table) does she imitate you? ○

32. Does she look to other children and imitate what they do? ○

33. Does she like to *be* with other children although not playing *with* them? ○

34. Can she join in when playing with older children? ○

35. Is it easier to leave her, and is she now a little happier when with strangers? ○

36. Does she hug and carry a doll or soft toy? ○

37. Does she show off? ○

38. Will she give you a book to read to her or the remote control to switch on the TV? ○

39. Does she pull at your clothes when she wants to show you something? ○

40. Does she say 'NO!' or 'HOT!' if she is near to something she must not touch? ○

41. Does she greet you? ○

42. Does she greet her friends? ○

43. Does she do as she's told at least half of the time? ○

44. Does she say please and thank you if reminded? ○

45. Does she try to be helpful? ○

46. Does she have tantrums? ○

47. After a tantrum does she quickly recover so it is as if nothing has happened? ○

48. Does she like to dress up? ○

49. Does she pretend? ○

50. Will she make a choice if you ask? ○

51. Does she understand the words 'love' and 'angry'? ○

52. Does she sing and/or dance? ○

53. Does she say 'Hello' without being asked? ○

54. Can she follow rules? ○

55. Does she ask permission? ○

56. Does she talk on the phone? ○

57. Can she follow a game with rules, such as Snakes and Ladders or Snap? ○

58. Does she do as she is told most of the time (around 75%)? ○

59. Do you have more warning that she is about to have a tantrum? ○

60. Is she upset after she has had a tantrum? ○

61. Does she have fewer tantrums than she did six months ago? ○

62. At nursery or at home does she chat to others as she plays? ○

63. Does she ask for help? ○

64. Does she join in family conversations? ○

65. Is she helpful? ○

66. Does she know some nursery rhymes? ○

67. Does she like you to read family stories? ○

68. Does she enjoy the company of other children? ○

69. Does she play exuberant games with other children? ○

70. Does she know how to behave in public? ○

71. Have tantrums disappeared or become more of a rarity? ○

72. Does she ask permission before using others' things (at least 75% of the time)? ○

73. Does she say how she feels? ○

74. Does she explain to other children how the game should be played? ○

75. Does she join in the conversation at the dinner table? ○

KEY

The average baby will have completed the first 36 items in the first year, and item 70 by the time she is five years old. The breakdown is as follows:

1–6	by month three
7–13	by month six
14–30	by one year
31–52	by two years
53–57	by three years
58–62	by four years
63–75	by five+ years

Checklist for eating

To carry out this test simply tick everything your child can do. Since the list is constructed in approximately the order in which behaviours develop, it can also tell you what she is likely to do next. Practice makes perfect and imitation and encouragement play an important role. So children who grow up in larger families, and in families who do not mind mess, often become skilled sooner. When you run out of ticks have a look at the key on page 164.

1. Eats from spoon held by parent. ⭘
2. Drinks from cup held by parent. ⭘
3. Feeds herself with fingers. ⭘
4. Holds and drinks from cup using both hands. ⭘
5. Uses spoon to feed herself with help. ⭘
6. Uses spoon without help. ⭘
7. Holds cup by handle or with one hand. ⭘
8. Uses spoon and cup at table making a little mess. ⭘
9. Sucks juice through a straw. ⭘
10. Uses fork to scoop up food. ⭘
11. No longer dribbles. ⭘
12. Stabs food with fork. ⭘
13. Uses paper towel to wipe her mouth. ⭘
14. Pours milk/juice from jug into her glass. ⭘
15. Cleans up spills. ⭘
16. Clears away her dish after eating. ⭘
17. Uses correct utensils. ⭘
18. Spreads butter on bread. ⭘
19. Sits at table and feeds herself properly for the entire meal. ⭘
20. Serves herself from serving dish – if someone holds it for her. ⭘
21. Helps set the table – correctly placing cutlery, plates, glasses and table napkins. ⭘

KEY

The average child reaches point 4/5 by the age of one, 8/9 by the time she is two, 13/14 by the age of three, 14 by four and 21 by the time she is five years old.

Toileting checklist

On average girls are clean and dry a little sooner than boys. There is some evidence that bed wetting runs in families. If you were late becoming dry at night it is possible your children will be too. To carry out this test simply tick everything your child can do. Since the list is constructed in approximately the order in which behaviours develop, it can also tell you what she is likely to do next. When you run out of ticks have a look at the key on page 166.

1. Sits on potty or toilet for five minutes.
2. Uses words and gestures to indicate she needs the toilet.
3. Uses face cloth.
4. Dries hands and face with towel.
5. Asks to go to the toilet – but sometimes does not leave enough time to avoid accidents.
6. Uses her potty (for both wees and poos) at least three times per week.

7. Brushes teeth – but not very well. ◌

8. Is toilet trained by day – has no more than one daytime accident a week. ◌

9. Washes hands and face with soap. ◌

10. Asks to go to the toilet in time to avoid accidents. ◌

11. Is clean and dry by night – most of the time. ◌

12. Washes arms and legs when in the bath/shower. ◌

13. Wipes nose if reminded to do so. ◌

14. Wakes up dry two days a week. ◌

15. If a boy, can urinate standing up. ◌

16. Blows nose when reminded. ◌

17. Brushes teeth properly – if reminded how. ◌

18. Washes hands and face. ◌

19. Wakes from sleep to use toilet. ◌

20. Wipes and blows nose without being reminded. ◌

21. Can bath herself – but needs help washing her ears and neck. ◌

22. Brushes teeth without reminding. ◌

23. Gets to toilet in time, undresses, wipes herself, flushes the toilet and washes her hands. ◌

24. Combs and brushes hair (even if long). ◌

25. Laces and fastens shoes. ◌

KEY

The average child reaches point 2 by the age of two, point 12 by the age of three, point 17 by the age of four and point 25 by five.

Checklist for dressing

On average girls develop dressing (and all fine finger skills) sooner than boys – but this is not written in stone – and those children who have older siblings willing to demonstrate are also at an advantage. Remember that children do not learn unless you let them try. To carry out this test simply tick everything your child can do. Since the list is constructed in approximately the order in which behaviours develop, it can also tell you what she is likely to do next. When you run out of ticks have a look at the key opposite.

1.   Holds out arms and legs when being dressed.   ○

2.   Puts hat on head and takes it off.   ○

3.   Pulls off socks.   ○

4.   Pushes arms into sleeves when asked.   ○

5.   Takes off shoes after fastenings are undone.   ○

6.   Takes off coat after fastenings are undone.   ○

7.   Takes off trousers (fastenings undone if necessary).   ○

9.   Zips and unzips jacket – but may need the zip to be started.   ○

9. Puts on shoes. ○

10. Undresses – if fastenings are undone first. ○

11. Hangs coat on low hook. ○

12. Unfastens poppers. ○

13. Puts on socks. ○

14. Can put on coat, sweater and shirt. ○

15. Can put on T-shirt. ○

16. Gets dressed without reminding most of the time –
but may still need help with fasteners. ○

17. Does up poppers and hooks. ○

18. Puts on mittens. ○

19. Unbuttons and buttons large buttons when jacket is
placed on table. ○

20. Puts on boots. ○

21. Unbuttons and buttons up clothing. ○

22. Puts bottom of the zip of her jacket together and zips it up. ○

23. Dresses completely, including front-fastening poppers,
hooks, buttons and zips. ○

24. Selects appropriate clothing. ○

25. Ties shoelaces. ○

KEY

The average child reaches point 7 by the age of two, point 13 by the age of
three, point 19 by the age of four and point 25 by the time she is five.

Top Tips

1. Set a family example at mealtime by using your cutlery, table napkin, etc, correctly.

2. Encourage babies to feed themselves, and toddlers to dress themselves, even if this takes longer.

3. Take the time to show your child how to put on her socks, shoes, coat and trousers. If you do everything for your child why should she learn to do things for herself?

4. Encourage your child to pretend. When she dresses up and plays at doing things that adults do, she is able to think about the roles others play in her life.

5. Parents are the central characters in a child's life. She needs to work out that we do not share her thoughts and feelings, and one of the ways she does this is to pretend at being the parent. Children need props that characterise parents in all their diverse roles – parent, worker, gardener, cook, housekeeper: glasses, high-heeled shoes, a drill, a garden spade, a set of saucepans.

6. Children should be encouraged to manipulate and evaluate ideas. When parents seek their child's opinion they help them understand that each of us has separate thoughts and feelings.

7. Remember that as children grow up they should feel free to express their feelings and opinions – providing they do so in an acceptable way.

8. Love her for herself, not what she can do, and when she behaves badly criticise the behaviour not the child.

9. Girls and boys must learn their gender identity: that they are, were and always will be female or male. But these days it is hard for girls and boys to know what it is that women do that men do not do – after all both sexes are now involved with the workplace, childcare and household tasks. All small children see things in black and white: in time they will see that although our gender identity is very different, in the modern world our gender roles are not that different.

10. If children play together, make sure that they also share outings and that they have the props to play pretend games based on these experiences.

Chapter 5
Testing Your Child's Temperament

It is Jamie's birthday party and he has invited all the boys from his nursery. As they arrive at the party each child behaves differently. Jack and Sanjay hand over their presents and race into the garden: Jack to ride the bike, Sanjay to jump on the inflatable. Sam is reluctant to hand over his present and then his father has to persuade him to join in with the other children. Alfie clings tightly to his father and asks to go home. Luke finds a corner by himself where he can play with Jamie's cars. Joe looks for Mohammed (his best friend) and for the rest of the party they are inseparable.

None of this happens by chance; if we had watched how the children behaved on their first day at nursery it would be rather like this and if we had watched them going into other children's parties it would have been very much like this. Children take a unique part of themselves into every new situation, a part that makes them act differently from other children. We call that 'unique part' their temperament and later their personality.

Before we had children many of us may have felt that life moulded children to be outgoing or shy, social or self-contained, but once we have children most of us are more ready to say that some aspects of their character were there from the start: and this is what research has found to be so.

Temperament is defined as those aspects of a child's mode of responding that are individual to a particular child and remain consistent between situations and stable over time. The 'aspects' in question include:

❑ Individual differences in emotionality – both in what we might call the child's baseline mood and the amount and frequency with which that mood swings from that baseline.

❑ Activity levels – how much the child chooses activity over inactivity AND what we might call the child's restless energy.

❑ 'Attention reactivity' – how easily the child is distracted from what he is doing and how easily he becomes bored with an activity.

❑ Self-regulation – the regularity of basic biological processes such as sleeping, alertness, hunger or digestion.

Are boys and girls different?

Despite society's expectations, there are remarkably few differences between the basic temperaments of baby boys and girls. Boys are more vulnerable to illness, have higher rates of infant mortality and are more likely to be injured in accidents (even when strapped into car seats, boys are more vulnerable to injury than their sisters strapped into the seats beside them). That vulnerability has a known cause: the male hormone testosterone. It is why men die, on average, four years earlier than women. If castrated, men would live as long as women, just as spayed tomcats live as long as females do. (I suspect most men would say it was not worth four extra years of old age!) The vulnerability difference is in any case very small. In as much as illness affects mood, vulnerability can affect temperament. Boys are often a little more active and restless but again it's a small difference and there is a huge overlap in the levels of girls' and boys' activity. There is certainly more variability between all the girls and all the boys than between the two sexes. In spite of society's expectations girls are not all sugar and spice and are just as likely as boys to be difficult. Nor are all boys hyperactive and easily distracted – although there are more boys than girls amongst the hyperactive and extremely inattentive.

Born with or learned?

Studies that have looked at the temperament of twins find striking similarities in activity levels, in measures of emotionality (the intensity of reaction, baseline mood), sociability (how readily they approach or withdraw from people) and in their ability to inhibit responding (a scale that includes attention span, persistence and distractibility). However, although something of what we are is probably there from the start, it would be wrong to think that this is the only factor that makes our children the temperamental creatures that they are. Life can also change us: things are not fair and we do not all start – or stay – on the same level playing field.

We know that early experience can change us because, if we look at the life histories of unhappy adults, the routes to that unhappiness and mistrust can often be found in their early years. To take an extreme case it is unlikely that a child exposed to physical and sexual abuse from an early age would be untouched by such experiences or that they could become the happy, carefree adult that their birth temperament predicted. But not every unhappy adult has an unhappy childhood. Sometimes there seems no rhyme or reason for a person's unhappiness (or indeed happiness) and for people like this we can probably say 'It is just the way they are'.

Although parents do not mean to, by giving children their undivided attention, they often reward and encourage children to do the very things they find least appealing. A boisterous child is shouted at when he races around, but ignored while he sits watching TV; a difficult child is 'tiptoed' around because we just haven't the time or patience to cope with the consequences of upsetting him at the moment. In time, his moods (or potential moods) come to control the family. We are more likely to give in to his demands than to those of his calmer brother because he will go 'off on one' if we challenge him. In our busy lives a child who behaves badly instantly gains our attention. When he is well behaved he is often ignored. It takes a real effort for tired and busy parents to act differently.

This state of affairs is likely to be more acute with a difficult child. A demanding, emotional and often unhappy child is more difficult to parent and we naturally relish the quiet times when we switch off parenting and steal a little 'me first' time. The last thing we intend to do at such times is to encourage his demanding behaviour! But logically it is often what we are doing. Small children cannot survive without us and need to make sure they are uppermost in our thoughts, that we care for them, protect them and keep them from harm. It is natural for them to desire our undivided and constant attention. If we give this when they demand, and withdraw when they are good, we reward bad behaviour and discourage good behaviour.

So some aspects of temperament are inborn, while some are learned (and how and what is learned probably interacts with those inborn tendencies). But that is not all. Temperament is almost certainly influenced by another factor: the child's expectation of himself and the family's (and later society's) expectations of him. Children do what they (and we) believe they should and expect them to do. In one experiment, children who were told they were really good at clearing up kept their rooms much tidier than those who were told – or shown – how to tidy the room. More surprisingly perhaps, children who were told they were really good at maths (even when they were not) got higher marks in maths tests than children given extra maths lessons. If it can work for maths, school abilities and health, think how it can work for behaviour. A child who thinks he is difficult is likely to become (or stay) more difficult. One who thinks he is easy-going is likely to become (or stay) that way.

All of this suggests that although the way children behave in the first weeks of life is often predictive of later behaviour, this does not mean that children do not, or cannot change, nor that the nature of the child is somehow writ large in his genetic endowment. The fact that many difficult babies grow up to be difficult adults is also a function of our (and their) expectations and the way we reward their behaviour.

The following test assesses your child's temperament. It is loosely based on a study carried out by Alexander Thomas and Stella Chess into the temperaments of a large group of American children who were followed over a period of many years. There are three versions of the test: one for babies (0–14 months), one for toddlers (14–30 months) and one for preschoolers (30 months–5 years).

Assess Your Baby's Temperament

1. Your baby kicked and squirmed a lot in the womb.

a) False.

b) True.

c) Neither entirely true nor false.

2. If your baby is awake he is usually quite restless.

a) False.

b) True.

c) Neither entirely true nor false.

3. If you pick your baby up he often squirms until you put him down.

a) False.

b) True.

c) Neither entirely true nor false.

4. Once your baby could crawl (or walk) he was always rushing about.

a) False.

b) True.

c) Neither entirely true nor false.

5. As a young baby he happily watched his mobile for long periods.

a) True.

b) False.

c) Neither entirely true nor false.

6. When your baby sits on his play mat

a) He will play happily with a favourite toy for a long time.

b) He quickly loses interest in one toy and moves on to another.

c) He can sometimes play with one toy for quite a long
    time – but rarely does.   ◌

7. Your baby gets bored easily.

a) False.   ◌
b) True.   ◌
c) Neither entirely true nor false.   ◌

8. If your baby is crying it is easy to distract him.

a) True.   ◌
b) False.   ◌
c) Neither entirely true nor false.   ◌

9. Your baby can sleep anywhere.

a) True.   ◌
b) False – he needs a quiet place.   ◌
c) Neither entirely true nor false.   ◌

10. Which best describes your baby's moods?

a) He is a smiley baby, tears never last for long.   ◌
b) He feels things deeply; he screams with laughter but also
    with anger.   ◌
c) He is somewhere between a and b.   ◌

11. Except when your baby is ill or obviously in pain he cries

a) Very little.

b) A lot.

c) A moderate amount.

12. Which best describes your baby?

a) Easy-going.

b) Difficult.

c) Shy.

13. When your baby hurts himself

a) He cries or whimpers but is easily comforted.

b) He screams and cries loudly and may refuse comfort.

c) He cries and needs comforting.

14. When your baby is unhappy

a) He whimpers and seems sad but is easily comforted.

b) He lets you know! His crying is intense and he is often inconsolable.

c) He cries, but he can be comforted reasonably easily.

15. When something frightens or upsets your baby

a) He is easily comforted.

b) He is inconsolable.

c) It is quite difficult to calm him down.

16. When you ride your baby on your knee

a) He laughs and quickly asks for more. ○

b) He screams with laughter and demands more and more. ○

c) He may be a little uneasy when the game is new – but then laughs and wants more. ○

17. When your baby is given a new food

a) He may pull a bit of a face, but tries it. ○

b) He spits it out. ○

c) He spits it out at first, but will take it if mixed with other food. ○

18. At about four months

a) He smiled at strangers and was happy to go to people he did not really know. ○

b) He was suspicious of strangers and would protest if picked up by anyone other than his main caregivers. ○

c) He was suspicious at first but happy to go to others once he knew them. ○

19. Your baby's response to any change in his daily routine is

a) Mostly positive. ○

b) Negative. ○

c) Cautious at first but then positive. ○

20. A noise will wake your baby

a) Only if it is very loud. ○

b) Most noises wake him. ○

c) If it is moderately loud. ○

21. Your baby is slow to tell you that he is uncomfortable.

a) True – he never cries when he wets his nappy and, although he fusses more when he is ill, he is still fairly easy-going. ○

b) False – he is very sensitive to a wet nappy and very unhappy when unwell. ○

c) Neither of the above is entirely true or false. ○

22. If your baby tumbles and falls on the carpet

a) He picks himself up. ○

b) He cries and waits to be picked up. ○

c) He may whimper but picks himself up. ○

23. It was easy to introduce your baby to solids.

a) True. ○

b) False – it was a long battle. ○

c) It was quite difficult, but I wouldn't say it was extremely hard. ○

24. On holiday or visiting friends or family for the weekend

a) He is happy.

b) He is unhappy.

c) He is unhappy for the first few days but soon settles.

25. Would you say your baby's reaction to new situations was

a) Accepting?

b) Intense?

c) Cautious?

26. Leaving your baby with a new baby-sitter

a) Has never really been a problem.

b) Has been pretty much impossible.

c) Has always been difficult at first but he is fine once he gets to know them.

27. Your baby often slept through the night

a) Before he was four months old.

b) Rarely, if ever, in the first year.

c) Before he was eight or nine months old.

28. Your baby tends to fill his nappy

a) At about the same time each day.

b) At unpredictable times.

c) At fairly predictable times.

29. Your baby's daytime sleep pattern is

a) Regular. ○
b) Irregular. ○
c) Not entirely regular. ○

30. Whether your baby is hungry at mealtimes and how much he eats is

a) Predictable. ○
b) Unpredictable. ○
c) Sometimes predictable, sometimes not. ○

Assess Your Toddler's Temperament

1. Your child never walks if he can run.

a) False. ○
b) True. ○
c) Neither entirely true nor false. ○

2. If your child is awake some part of him (a toe, an arm, his whole body) is usually moving.

a) False. ○
b) True. ○
c) Neither entirely true nor false. ○

3. If given a choice of activity your child would

a) Watch a video or sit and look at a book? ◯

b) Ride his bike or push his toddle truck? ◯

c) Play with his kitchen or 'brum' his cars? ◯

4. If left to his own devices your child would probably watch far too much TV.

a) True. ◯

b) False. ◯

c) Neither entirely true nor false. ◯

5. When your child sits with his toys

a) He plays happily with one toy for a long time. ◯

b) He quickly loses interest in one toy and moves on to another. ◯

c) He can play with one toy for quite a long time – but rarely does. ◯

6. Compared with other children of his age is your child more likely to flit from one activity to another?

a) No. ◯

b) Yes. ◯

c) Probably a little more than other children. ◯

7. When you show your child a book does he

a) Become engrossed? ○

b) Want to turn the pages quickly? ○

c) Want to turn some pages, but like to look at others for longer? ○

8. If your child wants chocolate in the supermarket it is easy to distract him.

a) False. ○

b) True. ○

c) Neither entirely true nor false. ○

9. If you take a toy away your child soon finds something else to play with.

a) False. ○

b) True. ○

c) Neither entirely true nor false. ○

10. If you say 'No' to him your child soon finds something else to do.

a) False. ○

b) True. ○

c) Neither entirely true nor false. ○

11. Which best describes your child's tantrums?

a) Brief and less than once a day.

b) Prolonged or more than twice a day.

c) Short but more or less daily.

12. Which best describes your child's moods?

a) He is happy and any upsets rarely last for long.

b) He feels things deeply; he screams with laughter but also with anger.

c) He is somewhere between a and b.

13. Which best describes your child's mood on an average day?

a) Calm and sunny.

b) Passionate and temperamental.

c) Shy and cautious.

14. When your child hurts himself

a) He cries or whimpers but is easily comforted.

b) He screams and cries loudly and may refuse comfort.

c) He cries and needs comforting.

15. In the morning your child is playing but you need to get him ready to go out

a) He protests but then cooperates.

b) He is angry and remains uncooperative. ○

c) He is sullen and uncooperative. ○

16. When you chase your child round the room or let him jump off the sofa

a) He laughs and quickly asks for more. ○

b) He screams with laughter and demands more and more. ○

c) He may be a little uneasy when the game is new – but
then laughs and wants more. ○

17. If your child cannot get his socks on does he

a) Get annoyed? ○

b) Completely lose his temper? ○

c) Sometimes react in one way, sometimes another? ○

18. When something frightens or upsets your child

a) He is easily comforted. ○

b) He is inconsolable. ○

c) It is quite difficult to calm him down. ○

19. Does your child get over-excited?

a) Sometimes – mainly when tired or with other children. ○

b) Yes. ○

c) No. ○

20. A noise wakes your child

a) Only if it is very loud.

b) Most noises wake him.

c) A moderately loud noise will wake him.

21. Your child will not fall asleep in a noisy place.

a) False.

b) True – he needs a quiet place and the curtains closed.

c) Neither entirely true nor false.

22. Your child is slow to tell you that he is uncomfortable.

a) True – he never cries when he wets his nappy and, although he fusses more when he is ill, he is still fairly easy-going.

b) False – he is very sensitive to a wet nappy and very unhappy when unwell.

c) Neither entirely true nor false.

23. If your child tumbles and falls in the park

a) He picks himself up.

b) He screams loudly and waits to be picked up.

c) He screams but soon forgets.

24. Your child's response to any change in his daily routine is

a) Mostly positive.

b) Negative. ○

c) Cautious at first but then positive. ○

25. Your child eats

a) Almost everything that is put in front of him. ○

b) Very few things. ○

c) He is suspicious of new food but will eat it eventually. ○

26. Which best describes your child's sleep pattern?

a) He goes to bed and gets up at pretty much the same
    time each day. ○

b) He still does not have a very regular sleep pattern. ○

c) He is usually fairly regular – but sometimes wakes in the
    evening and during the night. ○

27. Your child's daytime nap pattern is

a) Regular (or he no longer has one). ○

b) Irregular. ○

c) Not entirely regular. ○

28. Whether your child is hungry at mealtimes and how much he eats is

a) Predictable. ○

b) Unpredictable. ○

c) Sometimes predictable, sometimes not. ○

29. On holiday or visiting friends or family for the weekend

a) He is happy. ○

b) He is unhappy. ○

c) He is unhappy for the first few days but soon settles. ○

30. How soon does your child mix with other children he has just met?

a) Quickly. ○

b) Not at all. ○

c) He is fine once he gets to know them. ○

Assess Your Preschooler's Temperament

1. When at the playground does your child prefer

a) The sandpit? ○

b) The climbing frame? ○

c) The swings? ○

2. When your child arrives at nursery is he more likely to

a) Go to one of the activity tables and chat with friends? ○

b) Find a bike and race around? ○

c) Join the children at the playhouse or go to the book corner? ○

3. When you are running around does your child

a) Join in happily, laughing and shouting?   ○

b) Scream with laughter and race faster and faster?   ○

c) Is a little uneasy when the game is new – but then laughs and plays happily?   ○

4. While watching TV or sitting at the table does your child

a) Sit still until the programme or meal is finished?   ○

b) Squirm and fidget?   ○

c) Sometimes sit still, but never for very long?   ○

5. Does your child go to sleep and wake up

a) Within an hour of his normal bedtime?   ○

b) At different times each day?   ○

c) In a reasonably regular way?   ○

6. Does your child usually have a poo

a) At more or less the same time every day?   ○

b) At quite unpredictable times?   ○

c) The time is not entirely predictable.   ○

7. How much does your child eat at each meal?

a) Everything on his plate: a predictable amount.   ○

b) It differs from meal to meal and day to day.   ○

c) It's fairly constant but not entirely predictable.   ○

8. How easy is it to get your child to try a new food?

a) Easy.

b) Very hard.

c) Moderately difficult.

9. When your child first started nursery did he

a) Need a little encouragement at first, but settled very easily?

b) Make a lot of fuss and was very difficult to settle?

c) Need rather a lot of encouragement but settled within a few visits?

10. Does your child mix easily with other children when he first meets them?

a) Yes.

b) No, he finds meeting new children difficult.

c) He is cautious but he plays well with other children once he knows them.

11. If your child were building a pile of bricks and it fell over would he

a) Start again?

b) Kick the bricks across the room?

c) Try again if encouraged?

12. Compared with other children of his age how well does your child settle down to drawing, modelling with play dough or a similar activity?

a) He settles better than many. ○

b) He settles poorly. ○

c) He is about average. ○

13. If a child steals a toy your child is playing with and will not give it back your child will

a) Find something else to play with. ○

b) Grab for it, scream and refuse all other toys. ○

c) Protest and try to get it back but give up and play with something else. ○

14. Would you say

a) His cup is usually half full – he is most often happy and content? ○

b) His cup is usually half empty – he is often irritable and unhappy? ○

c) Neither full nor empty – he sits somewhere between the two? ○

15. How often is your child moody and unhappy?

a) Not often. ○

b) Frequently.

c) Quite often.

16. Does your child fuss?

a) Rarely.

b) Daily.

c) Quite often.

17. When on holiday is your child

a) Happy?

b) Unsettled, clingy and quite difficult?

c) A bit clingy?

18. When your child meets someone new does he

a) Speak to them immediately?

b) Cling to you and refuse to look at them?

c) Approach them providing you remain close?

19. When offered a new food will your child

a) Try it – and probably like it?

b) Refuse it?

c) Try it with encouragement but probably say he does not like it?

20. When going to a friend's party will your child

a) Run in happily and join in the fun? ○
b) Cling and refuse to let you leave? ○
c) Seem rather overawed and need a little persuasion? ○

21. If you call your child when he is engrossed in an activity

a) Unless you speak quite loudly he acts as if he didn't hear you – however many times you try. ○
b) He looks up immediately. ○
c) He responds on the second or third attempt. ○

22. If your child tumbles and falls in the park

a) He picks himself up. ○
b) He screams loudly and waits to be picked up. ○
c) He screams but soon forgets. ○

23. A noise wakes your child

a) Only if it is very loud. ○
b) Most noises wake him. ○
c) A moderately loud noise will wake him. ○

24. Does your child

a) Find it easy to get on with most children and adults? ○
b) Find it hard to get on with many children? ○

c) Find it difficult to join in with other children he does not know? ○

25. When your child is happy does he

a) Smile, chuckle and giggle? ○
b) Roar with laughter, and jump and shout with excitement? ○
c) Become quite animated, laughing and smiling? ○

26. When your child is sad does he

a) Look unhappy, whimper and cry softly? ○
b) Cry loudly and is difficult to sooth? ○
c) Whimper and cry but is easily soothed? ○

27. When angry does your child

a) Look cross and maybe shout? ○
b) Scream, shout and maybe kick or throw things? ○
c) Shout and stamp? ○

28. When he hurts himself (but not too badly) your child

a) Cries or whimpers but is easily distracted. ○
b) Screams and cries. ○
c) Cries and needs comforting. ○

29. Your child finds it hard to concentrate in a noisy room.

a) False.

b) True – he finds it really difficult.

c) He finds it quite hard.

30. When watching a DVD or listening to a story

a) He becomes completely engrossed.

b) He fidgets and loses interest quite easily.

c) He is sometimes but not always engrossed.

SCORING ALL THE TEMPERAMENT ASSESSMENT TESTS

❑ **Mostly 'a's. You have an 'easy' child.** Easy children tend to be calm, sunny and playful with regular biological functions. As babies, easy children are the first to develop regular sleeping and feeding schedules; they are easier to wean and ready to try solid food. As they grow up they are more likely to have regular sleeping patterns and eating habits. Of course, there are times when these break down – when they are ill or under stress – but when their world returns to rights so do they. Easy children have their likes and dislikes but they are unlikely to be fussy eaters and take new foods and small changes in their routines in their stride. They are usually happy and outgoing and their moods are rarely extreme. They respond well to change and are easy to settle into new environments. They are fairly tolerant of frustrations and quick to try something new. In general, they are happy and sunny with regular rhythms and a readiness to accept new experiences. They are perhaps the easiest children to parent. About 40% of the children studied by Thomas and Chess fell into this group.

☐ **Mostly 'b's. You have a more 'difficult' child.** Difficult children display intense and often negative emotions. They are slow to settle into routines and hate change. They are the last babies to adopt a regular eating and sleeping regime and are hard to wean onto solids or off the breast. Later they are likely to be fussy and irregular eaters, refusing to try new foods, and sometimes failing to finish foods they like. They are suspicious of strangers and uneasy in places they do not know. As babies they cry more often and more angrily and as toddlers they have more intense tantrums. As they grow up they are more irritable, intolerant of frustration and demanding of attention. Everything is felt deeply: when they are happy, they are very happy; and when they love, they love with passion. They explode into action like popcorn, they fidget when watching TV, they are restless in sleep. They are hard to settle, easily distracted and find it difficult to concentrate. They are the most difficult children to parent but studies suggest that when times are really hard they are likely to be the children who survive. About 10% of the children studied by Thomas and Chess fell into this group.

❏ **Mostly 'c's. You have a 'slow-to-warm-up' child.** A slow-to-warm-up child is cautious and often shy but, once he is settled into a routine or knows the people he is with, is sunny, happy and playful – but any change (moving house, starting nursery, going on holiday) is likely to disrupt those settled routines. Slow-to-warm-up children develop regular biological functions more slowly than easy children, but once those routines have developed they are less erratic than more difficult children. They have moderately intense reactions with more negative moods than easy children but fewer than difficult children. They are slow to accept any change to their routine, and can be unhappy until they have adapted to the change. They are harder to wean and introduce to new foods but less likely to be really fussy eaters. They sleep and eat in a more regular pattern than difficult children but, as babies, were slower than easy babies to develop that pattern, and any change in their day-to-day routines is likely to disrupt them, and to do so for longer. Their temperament is generally mild and hesitant. About 15% of the children in Thomas and Chess's study fell into this group.

❏ **Mixture of 'a's, 'b's and 'c's. You have an 'in-between' child.** Living proof that it is impossible to fit all children into a few boxes! Like 35% of parents doing this test, your child is difficult to classify. An in-between child is like an easy (or difficult) child in many respects but not in every respect. He may, for example, settle easily into a regular feeding and sleeping regime, be sunny and happy like an easy child, but tend to be over active and easily distracted like a more difficult child. Children are individuals and tests of temperament only tell us those behaviours that usually go together – not the behaviours that invariably go together. The scale actually measures a number of different characteristics. If your child's scores are 'mixed' you might like to see the area in which his behaviours fall into the three classifications above. The questions relating to each characteristic are listed below.

LOOKING IN DETAIL AT THE TEMPERAMENT TESTS

	Baby	Toddler	Preschooler
Activity level	Q 1–4	Q 1–4	Q 1–4
Rhythmicity	Q 27–30	Q 26–28	Q 5–7
Approach–withdrawal	Q 17–19	Q 29–30	Q 8–10
Adaptability	Q 23–26	Q 24–25	Q 17–20
Threshold of responsiveness	Q 20–22	Q 20–23	Q 21–24
Intensity of reaction	Q 13–16	Q 14–19	Q 28–30
Quality of mood	Q 10–12	Q 11–13	Q14–16
Distractibility	Q 8–9	Q 8–10	Q 25–27
Attention span persistence	Q 5–7	Q 5–7	Q 11–13

How to use what you know about your child's temperament

Thinking about your child's temperament can help you to be more tolerant towards him, and helps you to plan the day so that frustration and upset can be minimised.

❑ There is no point in taking a very active child into a situation in which he needs to sit still and keep quiet if the situation can be avoided. If it cannot be avoided, be realistic. Take him outside to let off steam at regular intervals and make sure he has something to occupy his restless hands.

❑ A child who hates change will probably not enjoy holidays – so prepare for this by taking along as many familiar things as you can get in your suitcase.

❑ A child who is active and easily distracted needs the ambient level of stimulation turned down low if he is to concentrate – so have lower light levels, keep toys that are not in use out of sight, turn off the TV and radio. Such a child will almost certainly need to race about before he settles down to a calmer activity.

❑ A child who adapts slowly and withdraws from change will always need to be exposed to new experiences gradually and to be given lots of support and gentle encouragement along the way.

❑ If you see your child behaving in similar ways to you (but wish you were otherwise), the frustration you feel is probably with yourself: bear in mind that no amount of pushing, wishing, or encouraging has changed your behaviour. Why should it change his? Try to accept him as he is. Of course, it is always harder to parent a difficult child, and this is especially true if you are under stress or if you are feeling depressed or in a difficult mood.

From Temperament to Personality

Over the years researchers have disagreed vehemently about what constitutes adult personality and how this relates to children's temperament. In recent years there has been a general consensus that 'personality' is composed of five elements – usually referred to as the 'big five'. They do not map very precisely onto temperaments.

❏ **Extroversion.** The extent to which we engage the world or avoid social contact. Those who are most extroverted tend to be active, assertive, enthusiastic, outgoing and talkative. Those who are introverted are at the opposite end of these scales. Adults who have high scores on extroversion are likely to have been active children, with high scores on the approach–withdrawal scale; that is, children who tend to positively approach new places, people and experiences.

❏ **Agreeableness.** How warm, affectionate and compassionate a person is. The precursor to this seems to be more social aspects of the approach–withdrawal temperament scale.

❏ **Conscientiousness.** This is a measure of impulsiveness: impulse is the death of organisation so it's also a measure of how efficient, organised, reliable, responsible and thorough a person is, how well they plan their life and whether they are able to delay immediate pleasures in order to reach more distant goals. Do they save or spend? Do they snack or wait for dinner? The precursor here appears to be the child's distractibility attention span and persistence.

❑ **Neuroticism/emotional instability.** A measure of anxiety, self-pity, tension, touchiness, instability and worry; of how much a person's experience of the world is threatening and distressing. The obvious precursor to this is a high intensity of reaction, and more negative mood. Difficult children are likely to grow up to be more neurotic than easy children.

❑ **Openness intellect.** This is a measure of how artistic, curious, imaginative and insightful a person is and the breadth of their interests. It's a measure of the quality of a person's life.

Short-term Changes in Behaviour: Stress Scores

Some people believe that any major change in our lives – whether good or bad – can produce stress but most agree that the major stressors are negative life changes. When under stress even the most easy-going child becomes more difficult and vulnerable. Like adults, children under stress are more anxious, unhappy, difficult and prone to illness.

They become withdrawn, they behave badly and they revert to more babyish behaviour. For child and adult alike, the biggest stressors are major accidents and catastrophes, loss of loved ones – through death, divorce, or long-term separation.

Short-term separation is harder on children than adults. Adults find it difficult to cope when a loved one goes away, but they understand what a month or six weeks means. A child does not. To him such a separation can seem like a permanent loss. A switch from a much-loved caregiver, or a house move that takes them away from friends and grandparents, also produces stress, as does a change in parental work patterns that means the child sees less of that parent during the week. Other changes that can be stressful to children include the arrival of a new baby, a parent taking a new partner, illness, moving house and the 'second-hand' stress of worried and distracted parents. The worry, distraction or depression of a parent under stress or coping with an illness (their own or that of a loved one) brings about a different sort of separation. Background stress is added to in the form of daily hassles such as missing the bus, breaking a favourite toy, not getting his socks on properly, getting stuck in a traffic jam, etc.

Assessing your child's stress level and your own

Score **15** for the death of a parent in the last year, **10** for all other major stressors (including the death of a parent in the last two years) and **5** for any moderate stressors in the last six months. Add **2** for every minor stress in the last week and **1** for every five things that have gone wrong for the child today (getting a shoe on the wrong foot, spilling his milk, not being able to get a puzzle piece in, having a tantrum, falling over, having to go out when he does not want to, etc). Check your child's total score against the guide on page 206.

CHILD'S STRESS SCORE

Major	Moderate	Minor
Death of parent	Parent has new partner	Weaning
Divorce or separation of parents	Change of caregiver	Holiday
Death of close family or friend	New baby	Christmas
Non-resident parent moves away	Parent starts work	Starts nursery
Major illness of parent	Parents arguing more	Potty training
Major illness of child	Illness of child	Sibling goes to school
Depression/major stress of parent	Moving house	Death of pet

Child's score: _____

Score **15** for the death of a spouse or a child in the last year, **10** in a previous year, **10** for all other major stressors in the last year and **5** for moderate stressors in the last six months. Add **2** for each recent minor stressor and **1** for every five things that have gone wrong for you today (burning the dinner, getting stuck in a traffic jam, not being able to find your car keys, waiting on the phone, snagging your tights, someone being rude to you, etc). Check your score overleaf.

PARENT'S STRESS SCORE

Major	Moderate	Minor
Death of spouse or child	Starting work/change of work	Moving <30 miles
Divorce or separation	New relationship	Holiday
Death of close family or friend	Pregnancy/new baby	Family quarrels
Marriage	Arguing more with partner	Falling out with friends
Major illness of child or partner	Moving > 30 miles	Christmas
Major illness of self	Losing job	Worries at work
Clinical depression	Financial worries	Death of pet
Loss of job	Partner loses job	Take out loan

Your score: _____

WHAT THE SCORES MEAN

Score	In Crisis?	Stress	Probability of Illness
Score under 15	No problems	Low	0–10%
Score 15–20	Mild life crisis	Moderate	33%
Score 20–29	Moderate life crisis	High	50%
Score 30 plus	Major life crisis	Severe	80%

The likelihood of illness has been included in the box to give some idea of the negative effects of stress on you or your child. As you can see in the table a major life crisis leaves us wide open to infection. The fact that the hassles of the day increase our stress score alerts us to the interaction between stress and the child's mood and between our stress and our mood; also to the fact that, once we both get into negative moods, each of us produce hassles for the other. It's a downward spiral we need to learn to avoid. Because, as adults, we have more control over our behaviour – and only indirectly influence his – we need to put on a smiley face, let off a little steam and try to get ourselves back into the positive. If we do, we will probably draw him up with us: but it is easier said than done.

Top Tips

1. Love him for himself – not what he can do.

2. Make sure your child has let off steam before any sedentary activity. All children build up a need to race around and shout – and this is particularly so for very active children.

3. Remove distractions – if a child is easily distracted he will flit from activity to activity.

4. Turn down the noise. A child who is easily distracted cannot concentrate when the TV is blaring.

5. Always find something good to say if he has made an effort.

6. Let him know how proud you are that he has tried his best.

7. Provide challenges so that he can feel the boost of self-esteem that success brings.

8. Choose challenges for a temperamental child that carry a minimum risk of failure. If he constantly fails, his self-esteem will plummet.

9. Do not build up the importance of success before he has attempted the activity. He is more likely to feel deflated by failure if he feels it is vital that he succeeds.

10. Enable him: let him try, avoid over-protectiveness and expect good behaviour. If you tiptoe around his difficulties you label him as a 'difficult child'.

Chapter 6
The Parenting Tests

Parenting is one of the hardest jobs we will ever do. Fortunately it is also one of the most rewarding. There are times when our children frustrate us, times when they scare us, times when they fill us with love and happiness, and – let's be honest – there are times when we want to shout, 'It was never meant to be like this!' One thing is certain: they tug at our heartstrings in a way we could never have imagined until they were born.

This last chapter is about parenting. What sort of parent are you? What sort of decisions do you make? How in tune are you and your partner? You may each want to do the tests separately and see how you agree or just assess how you are doing.

The Tricky Situation Test

For the following six questions, tick which answer you are most likely to do or say to your child in each tricky situation.

1. You find your child cleaning the toilet with a toothbrush.

a) 'That's exciting! Why not come and play with some water at the sink instead.' ⭕

b) 'That is naughty and dirty. You will get germs and be ill. Come here and let me give your hands a good clean.' ⭕

c) 'Stop that now.' ⭕

d) It would depend. If the toilet were clean I'd probably just laugh. If it were dirty I would probably shout. ⭕

2. You discover your child playing with your make-up.

a) 'Looks like you're having fun, but let's get out the felt tips and do some drawing instead.' ⭕

b) 'Those are mine. Make-up isn't a toy. Stop that now.' ⭕

c) 'Stop that now.' ⭕

d) It would probably depend how I felt and whether the make-up was new. I might laugh it off or then again I might shout. ⭕

3. Your child wants to stamp in a puddle.

a) 'That's a good game but it would be better if you had your wellies on.' ⭕

b) 'Stop it, you are getting your shoes and socks wet. You can only stamp if you have your wellies on.' ⭕

c) 'Stop that at once.' ⭕

d) I would let her play if we were on our way home and not in a hurry. I'd grab her and carry her away if we needed to be somewhere else quickly. ○

4. Yet again your child is drawing on the wall with a felt tip.

a) 'That's a pretty picture but if you draw it on paper we can send it to Grandma.' ○

b) 'Stop. You know that is a naughty thing to do. Mummy's walls are not for drawing on.' ○

c) 'Stop that now.' ○

d) She does it so often it is not worth making too much fuss any more. So if it were where she has drawn before I'd let it go. If it were somewhere new I would shout, smack her or move her away. ○

5. You have just dressed your child in a clean dress and she wants to play in the sandpit.

a) 'That's fine but put an overall on.' ○

b) 'We have just changed your dress. You can play in the sandpit tomorrow.' ○

c) 'NO, you can't play in the sand in your nice dress.' ○

d) I'd probably tell her not to get her dress dirty and then be cross with her if she did. ○

6. Your child leaves the table with sticky fingers. Would you

a) Not notice. I don't think it matters. ⭕

b) Say, 'Let's wash your hands before you play.' ⭕

c) Say, 'How have you got in such a mess?' and wash her hands. ⭕

d) I probably wouldn't notice until her sticky fingerprints were all over the sofa. Then I'd shout. ⭕

SCORING THE TEST

Count up the number of a, b, c and d scores and put them here:

a............ b............ c............ d............

INTERPRETING THE SCORES

Democratic parents have mostly **a** scores; authoritative parents mostly **b** scores; authoritarian parents mostly **c** scores; and inconsistent parents mostly **d** scores. The parenting styles and their outcomes are discussed below.

WHY WE DO WHAT WE DO

We learn our parenting skills at our parents' knees, and if they were cold and rejecting, openness and acceptance may not come easily to us. Little children are very poor mind-readers: they believe what is before their eyes and ears. Kissing and cuddling may not come very naturally (and not all children want lots of cuddles) but words and smiles cost little. Make it a rule that you find two nice things to say to her for each criticism you make; that you catch her eye and smile more often than comes naturally; and that, however she behaves and however you feel, you remember to say 'You are my very special girl' at least once a day.

While acceptance fills your child's needs, consistency meets yours.

❑ A child who is unsure about love craves attention – and naughtiness is always the best way to get it. Children want to be loved, and they want to be the centre of our world. A child who feels unloved (whether or not that feeling has any basis) will strive to be at the centre, whatever the cost. She will prefer your bad temper (even your smacks) to being ignored. If you shout 'If you don't stop that now you will get a slap' and then say it again and again, she will go on being naughty until she gets that smack because all the time that she is behaving badly she is the centre of your attention. It is worth the eventual smack!

❑ You must say what you mean and act on what you say if you are to control naughtiness. This is where consistency comes in. If she craves attention the best punishment is for you to ignore her and walk away.

❑ If you give attention to procrastination she will always find an excuse not to do as you ask. Once she understands that procrastination is ineffective in gaining your attention she will stop.

❑ If you say what you mean and mean what you say EVERY time, she will soon learn to do things first time. Threatening – especially making continuous threats – just gives the child additional attention.

Have a look back over the test and ask yourself what a child learns in each scenario. The answers are something like this:

❑ **Answer a** Here is something else you can do that I will be more interested in. Here is a better way of getting my attention.

❑ **Answer b** Here is the rule that, if you obey it, will get you my attention. These are your limits. This is what you must do, and if you do not do as I ask we will fall out. This means I will ignore you and if you persist you will be punished.

❑ **Answer c** This is what you have to do. Expect to be punished if you disobey.

❑ **Answer d** It might get a laugh and it might get a slap. I challenge you to find the rule that predicts which one! This, of course, you cannot do because the rule isn't a rule, but a whim. How you act depends upon your mood, not the child's behaviour, and the child is left not knowing what she should do.

The Parenting Style Questionnaire

1. One of the greatest joys of parenthood is watching children grow and change.

a) Strongly agree. ○

b) Agree. ○

c) Disagree. ○

d) Strongly disagree. ○

2. There is always a right way to behave, whatever the situation.

a) Strongly agree. ○

b) Agree. ○

c) Disagree. ○

d) Strongly disagree. ○

3. I never threaten a punishment I would not carry out.

a) Strongly agree. ○

b) Agree. ○

c) Disagree. ○

d) Strongly disagree. ○

4. It is hard, but sometimes we need to make love conditional on good behaviour.

a) Strongly agree.

b) Agree.

c) Disagree.

d) Strongly disagree.

5. Teaching children right from wrong is the most important job of any parent.

a) Strongly agree.

b) Agree.

c) Disagree.

d) Strongly disagree.

6. Children need a consistent and predictable home life if they are to become well-balanced adults.

a) Strongly agree.

b) Agree.

c) Disagree.

d) Strongly disagree.

7. A child should be able to rely on her parents to empathise with her needs.

a) Strongly agree.

b) Agree. ○

c) Disagree. ○

d) Strongly disagree. ○

9. Children must respect authority.

a) Strongly agree. ○

b) Agree. ○

c) Disagree. ○

d) Strongly disagree. ○

9. When it comes to disciplining children, consistency is more important than anything else.

a) Strongly agree. ○

b) Agree. ○

c) Disagree. ○

d) Strongly disagree. ○

10. The joy of parenthood is sometimes overrated.

a) Strongly agree. ○

b) Agree. ○

c) Disagree. ○

d) Strongly disagree. ○

11. There is always something new to learn about parenting.

a) Strongly agree.

b) Agree.

c) Disagree.

d) Strongly disagree.

12. Children need to know where they stand.

a) Strongly agree.

b) Agree.

c) Disagree.

d) Strongly disagree.

13. I have had to sacrifice many of my life goals in order to have children.

a) Strongly agree.

b) Agree.

c) Disagree.

d) Strongly disagree.

14. Parents cannot be held responsible for the way their children turn out.

a) Strongly agree.

b) Agree.

c) Disagree.

d) Strongly disagree.

15. There are lots of people I could trust to care for my children.

a) Strongly agree. ○

b) Agree. ○

c) Disagree. ○

d) Strongly disagree. ○

16. Children cannot learn by their mistakes if we always rush in to help.

a) Strongly agree. ○

b) Agree. ○

c) Disagree. ○

d) Strongly disagree. ○

17. If we praise too easily children will not try hard enough.

a) Strongly agree. ○

b) Agree. ○

c) Disagree. ○

d) Strongly disagree. ○

18. You need to be true to your nature. There is no point in hugs and kisses if that is not how you feel.

a) Strongly agree. ○

b) Agree. ○

c) Disagree. ○

d) Strongly disagree. ○

19. Ideally, every child should be raised in a home with a mother and father.

a) Strongly agree.

b) Agree.

c) Disagree.

d) Strongly disagree.

20. If she pesters enough I tend to give in.

a) Strongly agree.

b) Agree.

c) Disagree.

d) Strongly disagree.

21. A child should always know her limitations.

a) Strongly agree.

b) Agree.

c) Disagree.

d) Strongly disagree.

22. Bad behaviour should never be tolerated.

a) Strongly agree.

b) Agree.

c) Disagree.

d) Strongly disagree.

23. There is no point in having rules in the first year.

a) Strongly agree. ○

b) Agree. ○

c) Disagree. ○

d) Strongly disagree. ○

24. You should always let children know you love them and that you always will.

a) Strongly agree. ○

b) Agree. ○

c) Disagree. ○

d) Strongly disagree. ○

25. There is no such thing as an absolute code of right and wrong.

a) Strongly agree. ○

b) Agree. ○

c) Disagree. ○

d) Strongly disagree. ○

26. Making reasonable demands on children helps them to become good and considerate people.

a) Strongly agree. ○

b) Agree. ○

c) Disagree. ○
d) Strongly disagree. ○

27. Love should grow and change as children get older.

a) Strongly agree. ○
b) Agree. ○
c) Disagree. ○
d) Strongly disagree. ○

28. You should never slap a child except in anger.

a) Strongly agree. ○
b) Agree. ○
c) Disagree. ○
d) Strongly disagree. ○

29. Small children do not need routines.

a) Strongly agree. ○
b) Agree. ○
c) Disagree. ○
d) Strongly disagree. ○

30. Children don't know you love them unless you show them.

a) Strongly agree. ○
b) Agree. ○

c) Disagree. ⟶ ○
d) Strongly disagree. ○

31. Sooner or later you have to let go and allow children to do things for themselves.

a) Strongly agree. ○
b) Agree. ○
c) Disagree. ○
d) Strongly disagree. ○

32. Whatever their age, a child needs a regular bedtime.

a) Strongly agree. ○
b) Agree. ○
c) Disagree. ○
d) Strongly disagree. ○

33. I sometimes wish my child were different.

a) Strongly agree. ○
b) Agree. ○
c) Disagree. ○
d) Strongly disagree. ○

34. Religion gives children a basic moral framework: if we are not religious we need to find an alternative.

a) Strongly agree. ○

b) Agree.

c) Disagree.

d) Strongly disagree.

35. You should criticise the behaviour not the child.

a) Strongly agree.

b) Agree.

c) Disagree.

d) Strongly disagree.

36. Whatever they have done, it never hurts to say 'I love you'.

a) Strongly agree.

b) Agree.

c) Disagree.

d) Strongly disagree.

37. You have to accept that children cannot always behave well.

a) Strongly agree.

b) Agree.

c) Disagree.

d) Strongly disagree.

38. You cannot always stick to the rules: there are times when you need to be indulgent.

a) Strongly agree.

b) Agree. ○
c) Disagree. ○
d) Strongly disagree. ○

39. You should always find something nice to say about what they do.

a) Strongly agree. ○
b) Agree. ○
c) Disagree. ○
d) Strongly disagree. ○

40. It is important to teach children that it matters how they behave to other people.

a) Strongly agree. ○
b) Agree. ○
c) Disagree. ○
d) Strongly disagree. ○

41. A child needs regular mealtimes.

a) Strongly agree. ○
b) Agree. ○
c) Disagree. ○
d) Strongly disagree. ○

42. You need to put yourself in your children's shoes.

a) Strongly agree.
b) Agree.
c) Disagree.
d) Strongly disagree.

43. It is important to teach children that it matters how they behave.

a) Strongly agree.
b) Agree.
c) Disagree.
d) Strongly disagree.

44. From the very beginning you should start as you mean to go on.

a) Strongly agree.
b) Agree.
c) Disagree.
d) Strongly disagree.

45. I accept my children as they are.

a) Strongly agree.
b) Agree.
c) Disagree.
d) Strongly disagree.

46. I expect my children to do as they are told.

a) Strongly agree.

b) Agree.

c) Disagree.

d) Strongly disagree.

47. Rules are for breaking.

a) Strongly agree.

b) Agree.

c) Disagree.

d) Strongly disagree.

48. In our family we do not have many outward shows of affection.

a) Strongly agree.

b) Agree.

c) Disagree.

d) Strongly disagree.

49. Rules should be firm and fair.

a) Strongly agree.

b) Agree.

c) Disagree.

d) Strongly disagree.

50. I try to be consistent but I rarely manage.

a) Strongly agree.

b) Agree.

c) Disagree.

d) Strongly disagree.

SCORING THE TEST

Put your score for each question into the framework overleaf.

❑ **For questions 4, 10, 11, 13, 14, 15, 16, 17, 18, 20, 21, 23, 25, 28, 29, 31, 33, 37, 38, 47, 48, 50:**

Score 0 if you strongly agree

Score 1 if you agree

Score 2 if you disagree

Score 3 if you strongly disagree

❑ **For questions 1, 2, 3, 5, 6, 7, 8, 9, 12, 19, 22, 24, 26, 27, 30, 32, 34, 35, 36, 39, 40, 41, 42, 43, 44, 45, 46, 49:**

Score 3 if you strongly agree

Score 2 if you agree

Score 1 if you disagree

Score 0 if you strongly disagree

PUT THE SCORES FOR EACH QUESTION INTO
THE FRAMEWORK BELOW:

A list	B list	C list
Question 1	Question 2	Question 3 ....
Question 4	Question 5	Question 6 ....
Question 7	Question 8	Question 9 ....
Question 10	Question 11	Question 12 ....
Question 13	Question 14	Question 15 ....
	Question 16	Question 17 ....
Question 18	Question 19	Question 20 ....
Question 21	Question 22	Question 23 ....
Question 24	Question 25	Question 26 ....
Question 27	Question 28	Question 29 ....
Question 30	Question 31	Question 32 ....
Question 33	Question 34	Question 35 ....
Question 36	Question 37	Question 38 ....
Question 39	Question 40	Question 41 ....
Question 42	Question 43	Question 44 ....
Question 45	Question 46	Question 47 ....
Question 48	Question 49	Question 50 ....

Then add the totals for each column separately and put them here:

A list score ......   B list score ......   C list score ......

INTERPRETING THE SCORES

The score is made up of two main components:

❑ The acceptance-responsiveness scale (list A).

❑ The degree-of-control scale. The degree of control has two sub-components
  • a belief in the necessity of rules
  • the consistency in applying those rules.

To get your overall score, you need to double your A score to make an accepting/rejecting score and add your B and C scores to get your permissive/demanding score.

You can then plot your score below. You should fall in one of the four quadrants as illustrated.

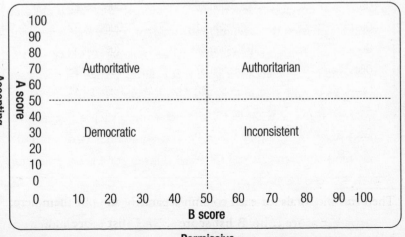

A high 'A' score plus a low 'B+C' score places the parent in the authoritative quadrant.

A high 'A' score plus a high 'B+C' score places the parent in the authoritarian quadrant.

A low 'A' score plus a low 'B+C' score places the parent in the democratic quadrant.

A low 'A' score plus a high 'B+C' score places the parent in the inconsistent quadrant.

❑ **Democratic parents** create a loving and accepting environment for their children. Children are treated as individuals and accepted for who and what they are. Although democratic parents have rules, children are encouraged to think for themselves and develop independence. Democratically raised children tend to be friendly, tolerant, independent, outgoing, active and assertive with high self-esteem. Democratic parents keep restrictions and controls to a minimum. It is more a case of *I expect you will behave* than *I insist that you behave*. When the system works, children do very well, but some behaviour (such as aggressiveness) needs to be kept in check and sometimes democratically parented children can be immature. This is not a good parenting style for aggressive or angry children.

❑ **Authoritative parents** are warm but assertive. Children know that they are loved but also that they have to behave. Such children can sometimes be over-protected and overly dependent, but on the whole it is a system that works well. If you have got things wrong first time around and need to get a child's behaviour under control it is certainly the system to adopt. While democratic upbringing can work well for 'easy' children, authoritative upbringing is by far the best system for more difficult children. The combination of affection and firm and fair control gives children security and high self-esteem and children parented in this way are often independent and high achieving. While less creative than democratically raised children they are also less likely to take drugs or drop out of school. Under most circumstances it is a recipe for success.

❑ **Authoritarian parents** set clear rules and get their children to obey. It's a very direct style of parenting that teaches children the accepted moral and social codes. It is not democratic; instead it teaches children to accept rules rather than question them. The up-side is that children have clear boundaries and know what to expect. The down-side is that it can make children socially withdrawn and sometimes sullen. Friendships are marked by argument and shyness and, as they grow up, children are more likely to be authoritarian and aggressive towards other children – sometimes bullying – or to turn their aggression in on themselves and become victims with low self-esteem.

❑ **Inconsistent parents** free their children from both the boundaries of rule setting and the mollycoddling of over-protectiveness. Children live and learn by their own mistakes. It's an easy style to enforce – especially for parents whose interests are often elsewhere – but not always an easy style to live with, either for the child or for those who care for her outside the home. The style fosters anger, rebellion and disobedience. Children tend to be aggressive and hostile and have poor relationships with their peers. It is not the parenting style of choice. Indeed it has been consistently found to have the most negative outcomes. However, many parents adopting this style are overwhelmed by other problems in their lives and many are suffering from depression: so we should not lay all the problems at the feet of the parenting style. For a small child, being ignored is the worst thing that can happen and this sort of parenting can be interpreted by the child as loveless and careless.

THE REAL WORLD

Although most of the time we all probably fall into one parenting category or another, few of us remain there 24/7. Under stress, distracted by things we must do and have no time to do, worried about bills or relationships, even the most democratic parent can become authoritarian and inconsistent. So what is important? Where should we draw our worst day bottom line?

If we look at the outcomes of the various parenting styles, two factors jump out at us: warmth and acceptance have better outcomes – and so does consistency. How you make and apply the rules is secondary to this. Remember, the most important outcome of our parenting is for our children to grow up believing:

❑ I'm loved without question.
❑ I'm worth it.
❑ I can if I try.
❑ It matters what I do and how I behave.

So our bottom line should always be that we put this message across. We need to make sure that they know:

❑ They will always be loved.
❑ They are very special.
❑ We appreciate their efforts.
❑ We expect them to try.
❑ They respect themselves as well as others.

The Parenting Test

This test examines a rather different aspect of parenting. We will discuss what it means after you have completed the test.

1. You fed your six-week-old baby two hours ago but now she is crying for another feed. Would you feed her?

a) Always. ○

b) Perhaps, if I felt she was really hungry and I was not in the middle of something. ○

c) Never. ○

2. Your six-month-old baby wakes half an hour before you are ready to feed her. You are making dinner. Would you turn everything off and feed her?

a) Always. ○

b) Perhaps. ○

c) Never. ○

3. Your eight-month-old wants to crawl upstairs. Do you

a) Block her access with a gate? ○

b) Sometimes allow her to crawl up but follow closely behind? ○

c) Allow her to crawl up whenever she wants to? ○

4. At 12 months your baby shouts for another biscuit. Would you give it to her?

a) Always. ○

b) Perhaps. ○

c) Never. ○

5. At 12 months your child wants to play with the electric socket. Would you

a) Block her access to the socket? ○

b) Say no and then block access to the socket? ○

c) Say no, and if she repeats it raise your voice or tap her hand saying no very firmly – but leave the socket as it is? ○

6. At 12 months your child wants to feed herself. You need to leave the house in 30 minutes. Do you

a) Not let her feed herself because of the mess she makes and the time it takes to change her? ○

b) Let her, but worry about the mess? ○

c) Let her, as you can clean the floor when you get home and most of the mess will be on her bib? ○

7. At 14 months your child wants to dress herself. Do you

a) Dress her? ○

b) Let her do the bits she can manage? ○

c) Let her try, and help as needed when she has difficulties? ○

8. At 18 months she refuses to have her coat put on when you go to the shops. Do you

a) Decide to put off shopping? ○

b) Talk to her and try to persuade her to put on her coat? ○

c) Insist that she is coming shopping – coat or no coat – and go without the coat if you have to? ◌

9. At two years your child wants to feed herself. Do you

a) Not let her because of the mess? ◌
b) Let her but worry about the mess? ◌
c) Let her? ◌

10. At two years your child wants to dress herself. Do you

a) Dress her? ◌
b) Let her do the bits she can manage? ◌
c) Let her try, and help as needed when she has difficulties? ◌

11. At three she wants to go on the slide. Do you

a) Go up with her? ◌
b) Let her go up but catch her at the bottom? ◌
c) Let her? ◌

12. At four she is in the swimming pool with her inflatable swimsuit/arm bands. Do you

a) Stay with her at all times? ◌
b) Go in the pool with her – but swim around nearby? ◌
c) Watch her from the side of the pool? ◌

LIST YOUR SCORES
1... 2... 3... 4... 5... 6... 7... 8... 9... 10... 11... 12...

INTERPRETING THE SCORES

This is a test about independence. Ideally you should see a gradual progression from beginning to end with more **a** and **b** scores near the beginning, and more **b** and **c** scores near the end. Good parents are flexible and enabling. They allow a light rein of independence throughout childhood, not a sudden rein when they go to secondary school or reach a certain age. You will have to stop feeding and dressing her before she starts school, and learning to get food from her plate to her mouth is always going to be messy. All children get their legs in the wrong hole of their pants and throw their socks across the room in a temper. So find ways to make things easier (place her pants so she picks them up the right way around, choose socks without heels so it does not matter how she puts them on). Your aim should be to gradually allow your child to become independent.

Checking Out Your Inner Voices

Complete the following sentences.

1. A good mother (father) would never

....

....

....
....
....

2. A good mother (father) would make sure that

....
....
....
....
....

3. A baby should never be

....
....
....
....
....

4. A child must always

....
....
....
....
....

5. I would be considered a bad parent if I

....

....

....

....

....

This test has no score. It is designed to make you think about the ways in which society, family and culture influence what you believe. Go through what you have written and ask yourself, 'Says who?' Who are these inner voices that are telling you what to think and, even more importantly, are they right?

The Co-parenting Tests

Test 1: sharing and expectations

This test is about you and your partner; what you think about the roles of men and women and about co-parenting. We hear a lot about the differences between men and women and their roles within the family. But what do you believe? And when it comes down to co-parenting how does reality match up with expectation? There are two sets of questions: one for each parent.

MOTHER'S QUESTIONS

Which jobs do you share with your partner and which do you almost invariably do yourself?

Expect to share   Invariably do yourself

Change nappies
Wash baby clothes
Dress children
Bath children
Put children to bed
Play with children
Take children to the park
Prepare food for children
Feed children
Go to children in the night
Find out about childcare
Discipline children
Collect children from childcare
Take day off work when
   children are sick

Score 1 for each time you expect to share a task but invariably find yourself doing it.

FATHER'S QUESTIONS

Which jobs do you expect your partner to do sometimes but almost always do yourself?

Expect to share   Invariably do yourself

Change nappies
Wash baby clothes
Dress children
Bath children
Put children to bed
Play with children
Take children to the park
Prepare food for children
Feed children
Go to children in night
Read childcare books
Discipline children
Collect children from childcare
Take day off work when
    children are sick

Score 1 for each time you expect to share a task but invariably find yourself doing it.

Now compare the father's score with the mother's. Do you have a disagreement? If so, go back and look at the areas of conflict. The point of the test is not to see who does most but to compare what you *expect* your partner to do, with what is actually happening. The final questions to ask yourself are how happy you are with the status quo, and how happy you think your partner is.

Test 2: do you share the same beliefs?

This test is about parenting ethos rather than practice. We learn our skills and our expectations about parenting from our own parents. We tend either to do very much as they did or, if we felt badly parented, we try to do better than they did. We do not share our partner's upbringing, and in many cases it will have been quite different from our own. Few parents settle down for a serious discussion of parenting practice in the months before their baby arrives. We go to classes about childbirth that probably extend to feeding and bathing, but rarely, if ever, consider parenting styles or beliefs. So here is a test that looks at your beliefs. There are no wrong or right answers here – or any scoring to find your parenting types. This test is for both parents – compare your answers to see how many of your parenting beliefs you hold in common.

MOTHER'S QUESTIONS

Answer yes or no to the following:

1. Should a tiny baby be fed on demand? ○

2. Should a baby always be picked up when she cries? ○

3. Can you spoil a baby? ○

4. Can you spoil a child? ○

5. Should children have a set bedtime? ○

6. Should children ever be allowed to sleep in their parents' bed? ○

7. Should they be allowed to come into their parents' bed in the morning? ○

8. Is it okay to leave a baby under a month old with a baby-sitter? ○

9. Is it okay for parents to go away for the weekend without their children? ○

10. Is it okay for mothers to return to work before the baby is four months old? ○

11. Is it okay for mothers to return to work before a child starts school? ○

12. Should babies be allowed dummies? ○

13. Should a four-year-old be allowed to suck a dummy in public? ○

14. Should a child be allowed to masturbate in private? ○

15. Should a child be allowed to masturbate in public? ○

16. Are manners and politeness important? ○

17. Is it okay to occasionally smack a child? ○

18. Should children finish the food on their plate? ○

19. Should children eat what the family eats? ○

20. Should children be allowed to choose what they wear? ○

Answer true or false to the following:

1. It is a father's responsibility to provide for his family. ○

2. It is a mother's responsibility to care for her family. ○

3. Those who work hardest outside the home should do less inside the home. ○

4. Those who earn most should have fewer responsibilities at home. ○

5. It is a father's responsibility to discipline children. ○

6. Parents are to blame for badly behaved children. ○

FATHER'S QUESTIONS

Answer yes or no to the following:

1. Should a tiny baby be fed on demand? ○

2. Should a baby always be picked up when she cries? ○

3. Can you spoil a baby? ○

4. Can you spoil a child? ○

5. Should children have a set bedtime? ○

6. Should children ever be allowed to sleep in their parents' bed? ○

7. Should they be allowed to come into their parents' bed in the morning? ○

8. Is it okay to leave a baby under a month old with a baby-sitter? ○

9. Is it okay for parents to go away for the weekend without their children? ○

10. Is it okay for mothers to return to work before the baby is four months old? ○

11. Is it okay for mothers to return to work before a child starts school? ○

12. Should babies be allowed dummies? ○

13. Should a four-year-old be allowed to suck a dummy in public? ○

14. Should a child be allowed to masturbate in private? ○

15. Should a child be allowed to masturbate in public? ○

16. Are manners and politeness important? ○

17. Is it okay to occasionally smack a child? ○

18. Should children finish the food on their plate? ○

19. Should children eat what the family eats? ○

20. Should children be allowed to choose what they wear? ○

Answer true or false to the following:

1. It is a father's responsibility to provide for his family. ○

2. It is a mother's responsibility to care for her family. ○

3. Those who work hardest outside the home should do less inside the home. ⊙

4. Those who earn most should have fewer responsibilities at home. ⊙

5. It is a father's responsibility to discipline children. ⊙

6. Parents are to blame for badly behaved children. ⊙

LOTS OF DISAGREEMENTS?

By far the best thing to do when you disagree is to talk about it. Sometimes matters of principle are just that and talking or putting principles into practice quickly reaches the compromise needed. At other times, compromise must be negotiated. It is impossible for a child to follow rules that are inconsistent: to do one thing when her father is at home or caring for her and another when she is in the care of her mother.

If you cannot agree about everything or compromise on strong and firmly held beliefs such as smacking or having children in your bed, can you prioritise? Can you give in on some points but hold firm on others? There is plenty of evidence that slapping may (and beating certainly can) produce aggressive children who are either bullying towards other children and/or the victims of bullies.

Children learn by example. If we get compliance by smacking so will they. As to sleeping in their parents' beds, most children around the world do so and come to no harm. Most American and northern

European babies do not co-sleep – and they come to no harm either.

Test 3: your opinions on the roles and behavioural expectations of men and women

This last questionnaire is about your beliefs about the nature of men and women. They are your opinions. The first section is for mothers and the second for fathers.

MOTHER'S QUESTIONS

Which of the following characteristics are desirable or more common in men, and which of these characteristics are more common or desirable in women?

	Men	Women
Attractive		
Emotional		
Loving		
Brave		
Seductive		
Good with money		
Decisive		
Accepting		
Intuitive		
Adventurous		

	Men	*Women*
Patient		
Clever		
Soft		
Hard working		

FATHER'S QUESTIONS

Which of the following characteristics are desirable or more common in men, and which of these characteristics are more common or desirable in women?

	Men	*Women*
Attractive		
Emotional		
Loving		
Brave		
Seductive		
Good with money		
Decisive		
Accepting		
Intuitive		
Adventurous		
Patient		
Clever		
Soft		
Hard working		

Again there are no right or wrong answers here. It is a matter of opinion. The only point of interest is whether and where you and your partner disagree.

Top Tips

1. Children have an absolute right to their parents' love. They should not have to earn it.

2. Parents do not have an absolute right to their children's love – they earn it by loving and providing for their children.

3. Criticise the behaviour, never the child. He is not wicked or stupid – but his behaviour can be both naughty and very silly.

4. Let your children know that you love each other.

5. Always be prepared to talk to each other about different attitudes to parenting. Do not assume one person is right and one wrong. If you have major disagreements it may help you if you talk it through with others.

6. The bottom line is that children need consistency.

7. Try to compromise and, if you cannot do so, try again and again and again. This is vitally important. How can a child understand if your messages are mixed?

8. Children have an absolute right to your protection, to your care, to food, shelter and protection from harm. They do not have a right to your indulgence. They earn that right by their good behaviour.

9. He is your child's father – whatever he does. She is your child's mother – whatever she does. You may criticise your partner to your friends and family but not to your children – nor should you do so within their hearing. You are the grown ups – and that is how you should behave.

10. No one can be a perfect parent all of the time: we are fallible and so are our children. Don't be too proud to say sorry and always kiss and make up.

Conclusion

The desire to help a child reach his full potential is at the forefront of most parents' minds. I hope the tests and little experiments in this book have helped you to better understand your child and, through that understanding, helped you to see how his natural abilities can be supported and enhanced. All children are individuals. Providing a nurturing environment for a particular child is one of the most important things we can do. Understanding the individual nature of each of our children helps us to do this more effectively.

The child you cradle in your arms in the hours after birth looks fully formed – and it is true that the bits we can see are all more or less as they will be in the adult. It is her brain and the thinking and behaviour it supports that is so different. Babies' heads are small and that means their brains must be small. Only about a third of the neurones in a newborn baby's brain are fully formed and many of the connections between brain cells have not yet been made. This means that our newborn baby sees differently, remembers differently and communicates and thinks differently. As the checklists show, the closer she comes to school age, the more like us she becomes. In fact, many would say that we have more in common with our two-year-old than the two-year-old has with her two-month self. It is time that produces the major changes, but experience also influences how the brain matures. As studies of those trained in childcare have shown, the best experience in which to grow and develop is provided by those who understand what their child needs. I hope the tests and checklists have helped you understand the individuality of your child's development, see the route she must take and how best you might support that route.

Remember as you go through the tests that the ages given here are guidelines. If an average child has just learned to do something it follows that 50% have not yet reached this stage. Encouragement and practice are good, but you must always work within your child's capabilities. Pushing too hard and expecting too much are not good for any child. It undermines his self-esteem and his confidence and this can cause him to switch off or to decide not to try. If you let ambition come from within, you protect your child's self-esteem. Remember that children who grow up in a loving, nurturing environment are not only happier and healthier: they also do better in life.